PICTURE PERFECT PRESCRIPTION

Also by Dr. Howard Shapiro

Dr. Shapiro's Picture Perfect Weight Loss
Picture Perfect Weight Loss Shopper's Guide
Picture Perfect Weight Loss 30-Day Plan
Picture Perfect Weight Loss Cookbook

PICTURE PERFECT
PRESCRIPTION

**An 11-Day Program to
Lose Weight, Add 10 Years to Your Life,
and Slow the Aging Process**

DR. HOWARD SHAPIRO

Chamberlain Bros.
a member of Penguin Group (USA) Inc.
New York

CHAMBERLAIN BROS.
Published by the Penguin Group
Penguin Group (USA) Inc., 375 Hudson Street, New York, New York 10014, USA
Penguin Group (Canada), 90 Eglinton Avenue East, Suite 700, Toronto, Ontario M4P 2Y3,
Canada (a division of Pearson Penguin Canada Inc.)
Penguin Books Ltd, 80 Strand, London WC2R 0RL, England
Penguin Ireland, 25 St Stephen's Green, Dublin 2, Ireland (a division of Penguin Books Ltd)
Penguin Group (Australia), 250 Camberwell Road, Camberwell, Victoria 3124, Australia
(a division of Pearson Australia Group Pty Ltd)
Penguin Books India Pvt Ltd, 11 Community Centre, Panchsheel Park, New Delhi–110 017, India
Penguin Group (NZ), Cnr Airborne and Rosedale Roads, Albany, Auckland 1310, New
Zealand (a division of Pearson New Zealand Ltd)
Penguin Books (South Africa) (Pty) Ltd, 24 Sturdee Avenue, Rosebank, Johannesburg 2196,
South Africa

Penguin Books Ltd, Registered Offices: 80 Strand, London WC2R 0RL, England

First paperback edition 2006

Library of Congress Cataloging-in-Publication Data
Shapiro, Howard M., date.
Picture perfect prescription : an 11-day program to lose weight, add 10 years to your life,
and slow the aging process / Howard Shapiro
p. cm.
Includes bibliographical references.
ISBN 1-59609-0529
1. Health. 2. Stress management. 3. Nutrition. 4. Mental health. 5. Excercise.
I. Title.
RA776.S4885   2005   2005041340
613—dc22

Printed in the United States of America
10 9 8 7 6 5 4 3 2 1

Cover and interior photographs by Gilbert King • Book design by Melissa Gerber

In memory of my sister
Marilyn Shapiro McLaughlin
November 18, 1955–July 20, 2004
Day after day, she showed me the true meaning of courage and
taught me just how precious life can be. Through it all, she had
the most genuine and gracious smile.

And for my brother,
Michael Shapiro,
in honor of the strengthened connection between us.

Contents

Day 1: Discover where your stress is.

Day 2: Is it chronic or acute?

Day 3: Complete a "stress trigger" inventory.

Day 4: Get in touch with the feelings that come from the stress you have.

Day 5: Learn not to catastrophize.

Day 6: Relax.

Day 7: Use positive self-talk.

Day 8: Think positive.

Day 9: Embrace pleasure.

Day 10: Feed your soul.

Day 11: Create something!

Day 1: Determine what shape you are in.

Day 2: What do you want exercise to do for you?

Day 3: What kind of exercise do you prefer?

Day 4: Make a calendar of your exercise commitment.

Day 5: Do push-ups to help develop upper-body strength.

Day 6: Do dips to further develop upper-body strength.

Day 7: Practice squats to develop lower-body strength.

Day 8: Learn how to do side lunges for lower-body strength.

Day 9: Do the plank for core-body strength.

Day 10: Practice opposite arm and leg extensions.

Day 11: Learn the power punch.

Chapter 4

Change Your Relationship with Food:

Day 1: Try something new.

Day 2: Focus on fish.

Day 3: Send for soup; hail to whole grains.

Day 4: Eat your vegetables.

Day 5: Strive for the ideal.

Day 6: Lower your risk of disease.

Day 7: Lower your calorie intake.

Day 8: Eat the pyramid way.

Day 9: Three-Day Healthy Low-Carb Blitz 1

Day 10: Three-Day Healthy Low-Carb Blitz 2

Day 11: Three-Day Healthy Low-Carb Blitz 3

Chapter 5

Day 1: How's your social health?

Day 2: Get ready to get connected.

Day 3: Assess your connectedness capability.

Day 4: Change the tape in your head.

Day 5: Serve your community.

Day 6: Campaign for a cause.

Day 7: Make a spiritual connection.

Day 8: Connect with the natural world.

Day 9: Be with friends; reach out to family.

Day 10: Join something.

Day 11: Do for others.

Chapter 6

Acknowledgments

Because this book represents a departure for me in so many ways, it is particularly gratifying to acknowledge those people who helped make it happen.

I must begin by thanking publisher Carlo DeVito, founder of the Chamberlain Bros. division of Penguin Group (USA), for spurring me to write the *Picture Perfect Prescription: Take 11 Days, Add 10 Years to Your Life,* I am grateful to editor Anna Cowles for helping me bring the work to fruition and for her calm and patience in helping me meet tight deadlines. She showed real grace under pressure. Thanks also to Penguin's Rachel Kempster for her work on publicity and to designer Melissa Gerber; each is exceptional in her field. I am grateful also to Meredith Phebus and Elizabeth Wagner for managing the editorial process and to Fabiana Leme and Pat Lyons for overseeing the book's production.

What is by now a team of people that has worked with me on book after book deserves my most heartfelt thanks, and I am happy to acknowledge my gratitude here: to my agent at William Morris Agency, Mel Berger, who guided me through this transition with infallible good sense; to Susanna Margolis for her help in putting often abstract concepts into concrete words; to nutritionist Phyllis Roxland, indispensable as always for her expertise and devotion to accuracy; and to Ed Claflin, the editorial magician who helped pull it all together.

Also part of the team are the extremely able folks at Dan Klores Communications—Judy Drutz and her assistant, Caitlin O'Neill, as well as food stylist par excellence Diane Vezza and her assistant, stylist Mimi Badgley. My thanks also to Gilbert King and Jane Huntington, the photographers who brought the food comparison demonstrations so richly to life.

At the office, I am grateful to Gerri Pietrangolare, Alexandra Lotito, dietitian Sharon Richter, and nurse Sharon Griffith—all of whom were essential to keeping my medical practice sound and strong while I devoted myself to this book.

Above all, I want to thank the distinguished experts who contributed so substantially to the writing of this book: psychologist Adele Fink, PhD, and psychotherapist Susan Amato, CSW, colleagues of long standing whose experience, training, and insights were invaluable to my own understanding; Carole Krupnick, who graciously offered her expertise in skin care; and those masters of physical fitness and exercise—Fred DeVito, Ron Fletcher, Michael Lechonczak, Heather Raymond, Lawrence Tan, and Yamuna Zake—who figure so prominently in these pages. This book simply could not have been written without them.

I am grateful as always to my friend Anna-Laure Lyon for bringing her unique sense of style to fashion-styling the book's cover. To members of my family—my sister-in-law Andee Shapiro, my nephews Jordan and Ross Shapiro, my brother-in-law Michael McLaughlin—I express my thanks for your loving support during the personal losses that so burdened the writing of this book.

Finally, my thanks to Kay von Bergen, who continues to exhibit uncommon grace in her support of my efforts at authorship and uncommon tolerance of my long absences and constantly shifting schedule. I appreciate her patience.

Chapter 1

INTRODUCTION:
TAKE ELEVEN DAYS, ADD TEN YEARS TO YOUR LIFE

*P*sst. Want to live longer?

You can! You have it in your power right now to add a decade or more of healthy, fit, vital, rewarding years to your life span.

What will it take?

Eleven days.

That's all.

In just eleven days, you can discover the lifestyle and formulate the patterns that will add at least ten years of fitness and vitality to your life. In these eleven days, you will discover a whole new range of possibilities, affecting not only the way you eat, drink, sleep, and exercise, but also the way you handle stress in your life and relate to others. At the same time that you're adding to your life expectancy—the years of your life—you'll also increase your sense of satisfaction, fulfillment, and happiness, which means the quality of those years.

In the pages ahead, I'll show you how.

I've been practicing medicine in New York City for more than a quarter of a century, specializing in weight loss. I know how to get patients to change their relationship with food so that they reach and maintain their ideal weight, satisfying their tastes while they eat the kinds of foods that stave off disease and add strength and vigor to their lives.

From Weight Loss to Life Gain

My patients have taught me that there is much more to health and vitality than attaining your ideal weight and eating a healthy, nutritious diet. Over the years, I've observed that my healthiest patients—the ones with the best self-image, the most vitality, the fewest illnesses, and the most optimistic outlook—combine four essential factors in their daily lives.

1. They know how to *chill* out—to get control of the stresses that drag them down. They have learned how to free themselves from tension in their lives.
2. They know how vital it is to move their bodies, to stay fit with *exercise*.
3. They understand that it's essential to maintain a *healthy weight* while eating nutritious food that tastes good.
4. They know that they need to reach out to others—to *connect* with the world in which they live and the people around them.

Not only do they know these things, but they have also worked out ways to put together all these life-expansion factors in their daily lives.

The truth is, these four life-lengthening actions are all related. Take the relationship between diet and stress, for instance. You can lose all the weight you want, but at the same time, you need to deal with stress. Otherwise, the health benefits that you gain by achieving an ideal weight can easily be wiped out by the harm of being wired, anxious, or a bundle of nerves. And not only that—as I'm sure you recognize, your stress level affects appetite, and appetite (of course) has an impact on how well you maintain your ideal weight.

Or consider what happens to people who exercise but don't take care of their personal relationships. At first glance, you might suppose that people who are really fit are the ones with the longest life expectancy and the fewest health problems. But not so. A perfectly tuned body will take you only so far. After that, researchers have discovered, the quality of your relationships with other people—in your personal, social, and spiritual life—has a huge impact on your health and your life span. You can work out at the gym till your body is an athlete's dream, but if you really want to improve your health and vigor, and extend your life span, you have to engage with other people.

Disease and Longevity

If medical intervention could eliminate the major causes of death in the elderly—cardiovascular disease, stroke, and cancer—how many more years could we expect to live? According to an article published in 2000 in *Nature* magazine, the absence of these major diseases would allow us to live, on average, another fifteen years.

There's Research to Prove It!

Fortunately, the essentials of longevity that I have just described—those cornerstones of life expansion—are now studied extensively by hosts of scientists, researchers, and doctors. I say "fortunately" because it means there is a wealth of evidence to support what I've observed so vividly in my medical practice.

In fact, science and technology have consistently extended the life span of the human species. When the twentieth century began, for example, our great-great-grandparents expected to live, on average, some forty-eight years. By the time the century ended, the average life span was calculated to be 77.4 years for men and 79.8 for women.

As I write this, in laboratories around the world, scientists are working hard to understand the process of aging, so they can perhaps find drugs that will slow, stem, or control the process— possibly even reverse it. It's not that we think we'll never die; it's that we want to live long lives with perfect vigor and keep our youthfulness.

Right here, let me give you an overview of what scientists know about the lifestyle factors that affect aging—and what every one of us can do to look, feel, and stay younger in body and mind.

1. Stress shortens life.

Incontrovertible research shows that stress drains energy, raises blood pressure, and reduces the ability of the human immune system to deal with invading microbes like viruses and bacteria. Clearly, there's a connection between stress and specific lifestyle behaviors—like smoking, drinking alcohol, overeating, being sedentary—that, quite simply, can kill us. With numerous studies in human behavior, researchers have proven that people who have the ability to manage stress live longer and better. And that's true whether you're handling the acute kind of stress that's the result of a major accident, loss, or disaster, or the more chronic kind of stress that saps your energy when you're tied to a hated job or trapped in a relationship that's gone sour.

2. Exercise is good for you.

Despite all that's been said in support of regular exercise, most people don't really know the medical reasons why it is so important. In this book I'm going to be very specific about the kind of exercise that can help the most with weight loss, staving off debilitative disease, improving mental health, and enhancing your sense of well-being. Fortunately, there is plenty of research to show which exercises—and what patterns of exercise—help you to feel better, live longer, and resist disease. The program in this book puts the emphasis on the kind of exercise that not only extends your life but also gives you new reserves of energy.

3. Eat right, live longer.

Eating right does not mean dieting. While everybody knows that health risks soar when you're overweight, what many people don't know is that the wrong kind of diet can actually shorten your life expectancy. The Atkins and South Beach diets, for example, may bring about immediate weight loss, but they have health downsides that nobody has told readers about. Both promote meat, poultry, and dairy foods that substantially increase the risk of a range of diseases—cancers of every description, osteoporosis, asthma, arthritis, kidney disease, and more. While both these diets promote unhealthy choices, neither of them offers replacement suggestions that would help compensate for nutritional shortcomings. In fact, the South Beach Diet offers no alternatives at all; its very rigidity is an encouragement to eat foods that should not be a part of a healthy eating plan.

What's more, these diets are strictly short term, which means people regain weight in a hurry if they waver from the prescribed plan. With Atkins—which has been around long enough for studies to be done—there is evidence that people who go off the diet not only rush to regain their original weight, but eventually go over the original weight. The metabolic process of ketosis, essential to the success of the Atkins Diet, accelerates the rapid weight loss, but it's not healthy over a long period of time.

Bottom line? *Such diets* will not do the trick in "curing" overweight. In fact, they *may actually shorten life and erode its quality.*

Achieving and maintaining *ideal weight* is certainly one of the most important things a person can do to ensure healthy longevity. But that's only true *if you eat the kinds of foods that actually advance health benefits.* That's why I don't subscribe to harsh, restrictive diets that end up depriving the body. Instead, I show people how to change their relationship with food. The result is that you'll eat till you're satisfied, enjoy the planet's bounty of tastes, lose weight, and keep it off. At the same time, you can maximize your body's ability to prevent disease by adding life-enhancing nutrition to your diet. And this can all happen at once. The program in this book will teach you how.

4. *Stay involved to stay alive.*

Some recent health research has stunned many doctors who held to the belief that pills, prescriptions, and surgery would provide the key to human longevity. It turns out that one of the key factors in long-term good health is your involvement with other people and with the world at large. Studies are conclusive: People in stable relationships live longer, are happier, enjoy better health, even do better financially than those who are more isolated or self-involved.

The interesting thing is, it's not necessary to have the most wonderful relationship with a spouse, partner, or close-knit social group. People who participate in any kind of cause— anything that takes them outside themselves and connects them to the world at large—enhance their sense of well-being. Perhaps that's not so surprising, since we naturally feel better when we're active. But it's been astonishing to learn how this enhanced sense of well-being both lengthens life and makes it more worthwhile. This is a critical link. People who watch their weight, exercise regularly, and take measures to control their stress levels may unconsciously ignore or bypass this critical component of longevity. Taking steps to overcome natural shyness or mix with people of similar interests may be just as critical to your health as controlling stress, exercising regularly, and eating well.

Sometimes it's all too easy to focus on yourself, particularly if you have a tendency to feel shy, housebound, or emotionally "not ready." But if you do that, you may be depriving yourself of an essential resource of good health. That's why this book has a program for initiating and sustaining this essential tool of longevity.

Whatever Your Age— Take Eleven Days *Now*

Perhaps you are in your twenties or thirties, feeling like you're at the peak of your physical and mental powers. Or you're in your forties or fifties, feeling much younger than that but starting to be concerned about your weight, your fast pace of life, and feelings of fatigue. Or you're in your fifties or sixties, quite possibly hoping for a change of pace—a healthier lifestyle, with less stress—but still facing many of the challenges that confronted you earlier in life.

No matter what your age, the eleven days that you spend on this program will pay you back many times over. These eleven days are not like a Caribbean vacation or a week at the spa, where you take a break and enjoy a completely different lifestyle, only to return to the same life you had before. The eleven days are nothing like an intense crash course or disciplined boot camp, where you have to follow the rules and obey the leaders. During these eleven days, you won't be dropping out to do something completely different—in fact, those around you may hardly notice the changes you make in your daily life. And yet, in those eleven days, you are going to have a unique learning experience. This is your opportunity to discover how you can smoothly integrate the four basic factors of life expansion into your daily life.

Let's face it. We all want to live longer. But the really important thing is to *feel more healthy, fit, and vital every day of our lives.* You don't just want to extend the number of years you're here; you want to stave off or avoid the decline of power and vigor that comes with aging. You want to keep your youth. And you can.

Longevity in 2150

The current betting is that by the year 2150, the longest-lived human could reach the age of 130 or even 150. This compares to the twentieth century's longest-lived human, Frenchwoman Jeanne Calament, who died in 1997 at the age of 122.

Claire: Dieting Was Not Enough

How do I know these four things can lengthen and improve life? Because I've seen it happen, and I've helped patients make it happen.

Claire was thirty-two when she became my patient. Already overweight, she was finding it more and more difficult to lose pounds. Like so many people, she had dieted time and again—and whenever she stopped dieting, she regained the weight she had lost.

With many of the diets she tried, Claire also put in the prescribed amount of exercise. She belonged to a gym, and when she was on a diet, she made an inflexible rule of getting there. But as soon as she stopped dieting and started putting on weight she would lose interest. Eventually, she didn't go to the gym anymore, either—the result of a complete lack of motivation. The result was that the only exercise she got now was the walk from the bus stop to her office.

I could sense Claire's tension the minute she entered my office. During the history taking, I asked about headaches, digestive problems, and sleep problems. Claire had them all. She also admitted to feeling constantly anxious. She tired easily, often became irritable, and had experienced breathlessness on occasion.

Her job just made things more difficult. Claire worked in a department of state government where she had significant responsibilities. She felt adequately compensated, and she had no problem handling the workload. The problem was quite the opposite, in fact. Her lack of interest in the job made it difficult for her to concentrate. On days when she came home most exhausted, she often felt as if she had accomplished very little.

These were classic symptoms of stress. With her sedentary lifestyle and frequent weight gains and losses, Claire was in a high-risk zone. True, she was only thirty-two, but I thought real change was necessary as soon as possible—before Claire began to experience serious ill health. The combination of stress, sedentary lifestyle, weight fluctuations—accompanied by a natural independence that kept her apart from other people many hours of the day—all added up to a profile of someone in serious danger. Something had to change.

Breaking the Pattern

Claire was clearly demoralized by the cycles of weight loss and weight gain, the periods of exercise alternating with days or weeks of being sedentary. She was fighting stress without any sense of control over it—and as her own self-image wavered, she went in and out of periods when she felt hope or despair about her marriage and personal relationships.

Claire had come to me for a weight-loss program. But clearly, that was only part of the picture. In the next few minutes of our meeting, I sketched out a program that is essentially what you're reading about in this book. All I asked was that she follow the plan for the next *eleven days*. After that, she could decide whether it was a program she wanted to incorporate into her life—or not. But even as I spoke to her about it, I knew that she was perfectly capable of breaking some of the old cycles and patterns if she would give the plan a try. She agreed to do it.

I told Claire that as part of the weight loss program I would be prescribing, I wanted her to join the support group that meets weekly in my office under the direction of a psychotherapist colleague. Claire was reluctant. She grimaced at the word "psychotherapist," but finally, with a shrug, she agreed to go along with the program, at least in the short term.

I advised her to begin a program of regular physical exercise, starting by walking, and if she could, join a gym. Claire promised to walk. With that, she embarked on my Picture Perfect Weight Loss Program, making a dramatic change in her relationship with food and in her eating choices.

A New Start

It was refreshing—and illuminating—to see how many benefits Claire discovered when she combined the weight-loss program with group contact. As the pounds dropped off (this time, for good), and Claire started to emerge from her shell, she began speaking up in the group. Others learned that she felt stuck in a loveless marriage and bored to death by a job that was little more than an escape from her home. What's more, Claire's personal troubles were more or less incapacitating her social life. She and her husband rarely went out, and most of Claire's friends had stopped calling.

When Claire started talking about ways to feel closer to other people outside her marriage, she seemed far happier with herself. Her tenseness and anxiety were reduced, and she worried less about appetite and eating than she had previously. Having seen how she could manage to eat sensibly, she also took charge of her exercise program—giving up the health club for a daily walk, which she enjoyed far more than weight machines. As her confidence began to build, she felt empowered to deal with other arenas of her life.

All of that happened in the first eleven days. Of course, after that, there was no stopping her.

Her exercise program, which had started with a walk around the block, became integrated into her normal daily life. By the time Claire had lost ten pounds, she was doing a brisk thirty minutes a day in Central Park. In a few weeks, her entire appearance was changing. The weight loss was noticeable, and the exercise had seemingly "lifted" her up: she stood taller and straighter and moved with more grace. Her skin glowed with color.

New Health and New Life

In time, with the support of the group, Claire made the difficult decision to end her marriage. She left her husband and moved into a new apartment; the move was disruptive but liberating. Perhaps stimulated by her new sense of freedom, Claire told her supervisor at work that she would quit if her job was not changed and expanded; she was then able to create her own assignment and moved to an assistant-deputy level in her department.

It has now been fourteen years since Claire tried the eleven-day program that changed her life. She lost thirty-six pounds, in all, on the Picture Perfect Weight Loss Program, and she has kept off the weight for fourteen years. She continues to enjoy brisk walks around Central Park, but now she has taken up running as well. Her second husband (of twelve years) often joins her. When the weather turns nasty, she does gym workouts in a health club near their apartment. Weekends, in good weather, she cycles along back roads near the couple's country home.

In her job with the state government, Claire rose to the level of deputy. But ten years ago, she left the public sector to start her own consulting business; this also meant she could spend more time at home with her twin boys. Claire and her husband are also active in local politics at their country home, where they are working hard to stop a proposed golf resort development they claim would pollute local streams and adversely impact the fishing that is an economic mainstay of the area.

Claire's tensions and anxieties went the way of her thirty-six pounds and her sedentary lifestyle—as did the headaches, digestive problems, and sleeplessness that were their symptoms. At the age of forty-six, she is more youthful than she was when she first came to see me at thirty-two. Her body is strong and slim. The only "medications" she takes are vitamins. Her life is active, engaged, committed. It is also full of stresses and strains, but Claire deals with those issues a lot more capably than she used to. With exercise, good eating, a loving family life, and engagement with the world around her, she is on a path to live well and contentedly for a very long time to come.

I Hate to Sound a Warning, But . . .

If you, like Claire, have been wrestling with the consequences of up-and-down body weight, stress, lack of exercise, and feelings of isolation, it's time to make a change in your lifestyle pattern.

If you can invest eleven days now, you can change your entire future.

Here's why: Think of your life span as you might think of your household budget or financial profile. Stress and isolation drain away your reserves of energy and work against your body's ability to fight disease, while exercise and a healthy way of eating are investments in longevity. Similarly, any yield from an investment in exercise and healthy eating can be offset by a loss of capital through stress and isolation. And just stopping the drain on reserves by learning to manage stress and engaging with the world is only that—a stopgap, not a proactive step into a healthy future that will yield the rewards of a vital longevity.

*All four of these initiatives together—**chill, move, eat, connect**—are essential for healthy longevity.*

A Look at the Eleven-Day Program

Over the years, I've refined and formalized the kinds of measures that worked for Claire and have structured them into the four programs in this book:

- a program for *managing stress*, source of the biggest killers in our society—heart disease, stroke, and related ailments

- a program for making *exercise* an integral part of your life—essential for maintaining vigor, peace of mind, and the looks that go with them
- a program of *healthy, low-calorie eating* that asks you to change your relationship with food once and for all—my proprietary Picture Perfect Weight Loss Program
- a program for *reaching beyond yourself* to the wider world and the people in it—a connection that has been proven essential for longevity.

If you tried to do each of these programs separately, it might take you months to figure out how to make the necessary lifestyle adjustments. But it doesn't need to take that long. With the eleven-day program, I'll be providing recommendations that allow you to address all four issues simultaneously in a very reasonable period of time.

The *first four days* of the program are about understanding where you stand in relation to each of the four life extenders; think of these days as awareness training. The awareness is essential. This isn't a matter of attending lectures and taking notes; instead, you will be playing detective about exactly where you stand on each of these four elements of longevity. You'll learn to identify your own stress-causing demons, to know precisely *why* you must exercise and *what kinds* of exercise work for you. You'll understand the principles of the Picture Perfect Weight Loss Program so that you can change your relationship with food once and for all. And you'll assess how you might engage with others for those all-important connections beyond yourself.

Following the four days of awareness training, you'll embark on a *seven-day action plan* for changing where you stand. For each of the four longevity initiatives—**chill, move, eat, connect**—I've structured a day-by-day program of action, assigning you steps to take each day and giving you the tools you need to execute the assignments.

Together, the four-day awareness program and the seven-day action program constitute a life-changing and life-lengthening experience.

What You'll Gain with This Program

What will be the consequences of undertaking this program? Some will be immediate, some longer term.

For starters, on the "immediate" side of the ledger, you'll lose an estimated seven pounds or more in eleven days. That is simply step one in changing your relationship with food so that you eat foods you love, eat till you're satisfied, enjoy the great variety of tastes in the world, and know that you're eating healthfully and for slimness.

You'll also seamlessly ease yourself into a daily exercise program. You'll get a handle on the stress in your life. And you will have taken the first steps toward commitment to lives beyond your own.

In short, you'll be slim, healthy, active, sexy, involved, and engaged now—and for a long life to come.

But the immediate results are only the starting point. By undertaking this life-changing and life-enhancing program, you'll have taken steps to prevent both the killer diseases we all fear—cancer, heart disease, diabetes—and the debilitating ailments that weigh down our later years—arthritis, Parkinson's disease, dementia, osteoporosis, and depression, among others.

You'll be on your way to staying active in body and mind for a lifetime. Think what that means. It means you'll always have the strength and eagerness to travel widely, to be on the move, to stay sharp and attuned to new events and developments, to enjoy books and movies and theater all your life, to be no burden to your children—ever.

And you'll look younger—more fit, more healthy, and more rested. That's the final promise of this program. The right nutrition and exercise, plus living a life that is as free as possible of stress and as rich as possible in connections, will show—in your body's slim limberness, in the condition of your skin and hair and teeth, in the strength you'll continue to bring to every activity, every interaction with others, every hearty handshake.

Think of the Children, Too

Even if this eleven-day program is just for your own benefit, it's for the next generation, too.

For the first time in American history, today's generation of children is looking ahead to a *shorter life span* than their parents enjoyed. Unhappily, they look it, they feel it, and they act it. Obesity has become an epidemic among American children, and diseases once reserved for adulthood are now showing up in teenagers and youths. Adult diabetes has become a kid's disease. So has elevated cholesterol. The children afflicted with these diseases aren't the only ones who will pay. We all will, in skyrocketing insurance costs, higher taxes to pay for more public health initiatives, lost productivity in the workplace—and, of course, the grief and despair of lives limited by disease or ended far too early.

The reasons for this disastrous state of affairs are all too obvious: fast food and supersized portions, even in school cafeterias; kids who can wield a computer or TV remote but can't walk a block without complaining; family members who pass one another like ships in the night, never sitting down together to a real meal; logging on while tuning out. Schools with no gym programs and towns with no sidewalks or bike paths. Pressure to succeed—in nursery school! From an early age, Americans are learning how to live unhealthy, unhappy lives. No wonder today's generation can be expected to have a shorter life expectancy than that of the preceding generation.

This new form of a generation gap was brought to my attention recently by one of my friends. She has always been an avid tennis player, and at sixty-one, she continues to enjoy the game as often as possible. Not long ago, she visited her daughter and son-in-law in Florida and played a few games with her eleven-year-old granddaughter. Before the set was half finished, her granddaughter was completely exhausted, while my friend, fifty years her senior, wasn't even breathing hard.

Unfortunately, my friend is the exception rather than the rule. She has remained active all her life. Too many adults, I'm afraid, have become sedentary, and that is the example that today's kids seem to be following. Systematically, we've thrown away or overturned the great opportunities for health and fitness that surround us. We've surrendered instead to the extrinsic and intrinsic forces that are killing us—from the competitive scramble and pollution of modern life to bad habits learned in childhood to today's popular diets. The effects of these forces are felt not just in the dread diseases we all fear—cancer, heart disease, diabetes, osteoporosis—but also in respiratory problems, joint problems and arthritis, decreased sex drive, gout, even skin problems, not to mention unhappiness and the high costs of health care. The bottom line? We're shortening our lives every day.

Diabetes and Longevity

Today, teenage children are contracting adult-onset diabetes—a direct result of their eating habits and sedentary lifestyle. What the impact will be on their life span can only be guessed at. But medical records provide us with the following clues: A man who contracts diabetes by the age of forty can expect to lose eleven years from his natural life span. A woman will lose fourteen years. Any boy or girl who has symptoms of adult-onset diabetes is certainly looking at the risk of a much-shortened life.

An Integrated Program That's in Your Hands

This book provides not an elixir but a plan. There's no expense involved—and no radical change in lifestyle. If you undertake this program today, you'll not only add more years to your life, you'll also keep your youth. Doing so is in your power. That means you're going to have to do some work. Here's why:

The aging process, as we all know, is influenced by genetics. But environmental influences have a huge effect. And while there's nothing you can do about the set of genes you were born with, there is plenty you can do about environmental influences. Making changes in that arena quite literally, and dramatically, affects life expectancy.

Take a simple example—one we're all familiar with. Do you smoke? On average, smokers lose fourteen years of their life to this habit; quit the habit, and you can start getting the years back. Quit today—no matter how old you are or how long you've been smoking—and you will immediately gain back a year of your life.

But here's another factor you can control, though it's not as easily recognized as a pack of deadly cigarettes. Is your blood pressure high? Many people don't realize that by learning to handle stress you can significantly lower blood pressure. Do that, and you can easily add 1.3 years to your life.

How about this one: Do you lead a sedentary lifestyle? Walk an hour and a half a day, seven days a week, and add a year to your life.

These are not fictional promises; they are actuarial assumptions used by insurance companies and based on years of statistics. They're for real.

This book will not so much concentrate on the bad habits you should drop—like smoking—as on four things you can do proactively, starting today, to achieve a healthy longevity. Actually, in taking these four life-extending measures, you'll effectively drop the bad habits anyway—virtually automatically.

The funny thing is, you already know something about all four factors that are part of the eleven-day program—***stress reduction***, ***exercise***, ***weight loss***, and ***connecting*** with others. We all know exactly how to live longer and better. Doctors have been telling patients how for years.

What I've done in this book is get it together. I've compiled the scientific know-how and the medical advice into a practical, workable program you can do in eleven days—four days of awareness training and seven days of action. In all, the eleven days are a life-changing experience that will give you a longer, healthier, happier life—one filled with youthfulness.

Surely you can take eleven days for all that.

Manage Your Stress

Awareness			
DAY 1	**DAY 2**	**DAY 3**	**DAY 4**
Discover where your stress is.	Is it chronic or acute?	Complete a "stress trigger" inventory.	Get in touch with the feelings that come from the stress you have.

Action						
DAY 5	**DAY 6**	**DAY 7**	**DAY 8**	**DAY 9**	**DAY 10**	**DAY 11**
Learn not to catastrophize.	Relax.	Use positive self-talk.	Think positive.	Embrace pleasure.	Feed your soul.	Create something!

Chapter 2

MANAGE YOUR STRESS

Why is stress management such an important part of the eleven-day program?

Stress is a secret saboteur that can take an incredible toll on your health. People who are constantly overstressed are at greater risk of a whole range of life-threatening diseases. *Put simply, stress shortens your life expectancy.*

But just as doctors have learned about the high cost of stress, we have also discovered many effective ways to *manage* it. And that's precisely what you're going to learn about in this eleven-day program.

In Days 1 through 4—the Awareness part of the program—you'll discover what's stressing you out, whether the stress is chronic or acute (they're quite different), what triggers your stress, and what feelings come from the stress you have.

In Days 5 through 11—the Action part—I'll give you the tools you need to gain control over stress, *including deep breathing, easy meditation, relaxation, positive self-talk, positive thinking, and other Picture Perfect Prescription methods.*

During each one of these eleven days, you'll be able to learn a little bit more about what triggers your feelings of stress. And from there, you'll discover practical, everyday methods that you have *within your power* to regulate, manage, and control that stress.

What the Experts Tell Us

In my own medical practice, I have been fortunate to have the assistance of two specialists who have developed remarkably practical and easy-to-use methods of dealing with stress.

Dr. Adele Fink, a psychologist, and Susan Amato, CSW, a psychotherapist, have worked one-on-one—and with groups of patients—on weight loss and weight control. Of course, these issues involve many psychological and emotional factors. Dr. Fink and Ms. Amato have helped create the stress-management program in this chapter and have provided me with some of the information and insights I'm about to share with you.

They know stress to be a consuming, exhausting, oppressive psychological condition that affects body as well as mind, damaging both, with consequences that have a grave impact on your life expectancy.

What are some of the causes of stress? I'm sure you're familiar with many of them—job pressures, an argument with your spouse, an endless commute in bumper-to-bumper traffic, money problems, accidents, divorce, deadlines, crowds, legal complications, travel, relationships with friends and coworkers. Stress is our response to these things; in fact, it's our response to anything that requires us to adjust to a change in the environment.

Interestingly enough, even people who have very high-stress jobs may be *most* bothered by the kinds of things that irk all of us. Not long ago, when I was guiding some members of the New York Police Department through the Picture Perfect Weight Loss

Program, I interviewed a number of them and asked, "What causes you the most stress?" I expected them to say it was their concerns about being on patrol, or entering dangerous buildings, or the risk of being fired at by some unknown gunman. But, not at all! They worried about the same kinds of things that are likely to bother you and me. One cop told me the big problem was that his wife worked a different shift, and because of their schedules, it was always a challenge to get the family laundry done. Here's a tough, big New York cop, and what's stressing him out? Doing the laundry! Another said he had a long commute from Staten Island, so his big stress was trying to get to work on time in all the traffic. In other words, the stresses that affected them most were the stresses of everyday life.

Do You Have Symptoms of Stress?

Do you have the following symptoms? How badly—and how often? If you exhibit some or all of the following frequently and/or with intensity, you may really be suffering from stress. Bottom line: A headache may not be just a headache but a marker of an underlying stress condition. The same for recurring diarrhea, poor appetite, dizziness, etc. Consult the chart on the next page and check off the symptoms you've experienced to get a picture of your possible stress profile.

Do You Have . . .

Symptom	Sometimes	Frequently	Badly	Not So Bad	Never
Headaches					
Digestive problems					
Sleeplessness					
Worry/anxiety					
Feeling guilty					
Feeling worthless					
Poor appetite					
Crying easily					
Loneliness					
Feeling fat, gaining weight					
Lack of interest or pleasure in sex					
Irritability					
Tiring easily					
Feeling shy or self-conscious					
Trouble concentrating					
Feeling tense, keyed up					
Irrational fears					
Faintness, dizziness					
Stomach ulcers, colitis					
Chest pains					
Nausea, upset stomach					
Recurring diarrhea					
Chronic constipation					
Sadness, depression					
Trouble getting your breath					
Feeling like you can't go on					

What Stress Does to You

Feel like blowing your stack? Stamping your feet? Venting your frustration? Those responses are not just emotional. They're also physical. Briefly, here's what happens when you perceive a change in your environment.

Your awareness of the change instantly activates your hypothalamus, the part of the brain that regulates body temperature, metabolism, and automatic response to stimuli. The hypothalamus in turn triggers the pituitary gland, causing the secretion of various hormones.

Your spinal cord's nervous system stimulates your body's organs.

Your heart pumps harder and faster, spurred by increased activity in the adrenal glands, and the speeded-up heart rate increases blood flow to muscles and organs and raises your blood sugar level.

Your breathing also speeds up, becoming shallower and forcing a greater flow of oxygen into the body.

Your liver releases glycogen to provide extra energy to deal with the change you have sensed, while your stomach and intestines slow down.

Your pupils dilate; more light enters your eye.

You get goose bumps; your hair literally stands up.

Your muscles tighten and strengthen in preparation for coordinated movement.

All of this happens in nanoseconds, of course—so fast and so automatically you may be almost unaware of it. And obviously, there is nothing wrong with these responses or with your feelings of fear, anxiety, and oppression; they are natural, normal, and an intrinsic part of human physiology. But if the responses continue repeatedly, or if you perceive constant change in the environment, or if the stress alert goes on past the action it has motivated or the new awareness it has generated, then the physical effects begin to be wearing. The resources your body spends on the stress response are resources diverted from their regular health maintenance tasks.

Good Stress

Of course, in addition to being *life-threatening*, stress can be *life-saving*. In the classic example, stress is what enables a young mother to lift a light pole that has fallen on her five-year-old child. All that adrenaline coursing through her body and all those heightened physical reactions it produced can indeed provide "superhuman" power.

Stress can also prove beneficial under more ordinary circumstances. Because it involves a change in the way we behave or approach events, circumstances, and occurrences, stress creates demands on us. It requires us to step up to the plate, to rise to the occasion. At the best of times, those demands and requirements can stimulate us to excel. In such situations, stress can energize and motivate us and is indeed what makes our lives exciting.

Here are some typical good stresses:
• A new job
• Marriage
• A new baby
• A book so thrilling you can't put it down
• A game of racquetball/chess/tennis/you-name-it against an opponent who exactly matches your skills and abilities
• A time limit or deadline

The Danger to Your Health

Research on the impact of stress on the body's immune response has found that higher levels of stress can reduce the cellular response to infection and can actually slow the process of healing from a wound—anything from an everyday scratch to a surgical incision. *In other words, stress reduces your body's ability to fight back against both disease and physical trauma.*

Stress shows up in the way you feel—in warning signs that range from headaches, neck and back pain, upset stomach, rashes, and sleeplessness to ulcers, high blood pressure, heart disease, and stroke. So when Dr. Fink and Ms. Amato are helping patients manage stress, they're also helping them avoid the many kinds of illness, disorders, and disease that are directly related to the emotional and physical pressure cooker. And that means helping people to live longer.

People like Barbara and Jessica.

Barbara: A Countdown to Trouble

Barbara's long days are shortening her life.

Her alarm goes off at four-thirty, and the car service arrives promptly at five. Barbara and her supersized cup of coffee take up a position in the backseat, where Barbara can work her Blackberry between sips of high-powered espresso. She's in the office by six o'clock, and she rarely leaves before nine o'clock at night. She has a large, competent staff ready to do her bidding, but the fact is that her job, exalted though it is, is on the line every day.

Barbara feels the responsibility right in the pit of her stomach. When her numbers are down and her division isn't meeting its targets, Barbara feels even worse. She is acutely aware that her predecessor was let go when she failed to meet projections, and Barbara is determined to make sure she doesn't suffer the same fate. But when she feels her job is on the line, she takes it out on her staff. They've learned to keep their distance. They're tired of being barked at because the boss is frustrated. She knows she's been pushing them to do things before they understand what they're doing.

Barbara respects the importance of exercise, and she has a treadmill right in her office. She often climbs onto it when she needs to make phone calls. She can power-walk and talk on the headset at the same furious pace. Her doctor has warned her about high blood pressure, and theoretically, this daily exercise should bring it down. But it hasn't worked out that way. Blood pressure is still a problem. Even weekend massages aren't helping her muscle tension.

Barbara is forty-four. At this rate, she'll be lucky to make it to sixty.

Looking for Relief

As a doctor, I can tell you that Barbara presents the classic symptoms of too much stress. Her blood pressure is high, her muscles are tense, she has chronic "butterflies" in her stomach. She is irritable and almost surely depressed, though she masks it with nervous agitation. There's so much stress in her life that it has affected her immune system, making her a target for infection of every sort, and she already suffers from reduced sex drive.

Even scarier, research has shown that the kind of stress Barbara is undergoing can affect cognition—literally, it can age the brain. More obviously, Barbara is definitely not getting enough good rest; her exercise "program" appears to be simply another way to work even harder and more aggressively. She eats and drinks too much on the weekends, even though she knows that these binges of food and alcohol are both mindless and physically harmful.

Until and unless she deals with the persistent stress, Barbara will continue to use up her physiological, psychological, and emotional resources on her way to an early death. If so, she'll be one of millions of people who allow themselves to be killed well before their time by the effects of stress. And even when the effects of stress are not life-shortening, it takes a serious toll—decreasing feelings of youthfulness, energy, and enjoyment of life today.

Jessica: Pressure from All Sides— A Massive Stress

Jessica is another patient of mine. At first glance, you'd think the problems of her life are far removed from those of Barbara. In some ways, Jessica is the classic soccer mom. True, she doesn't have to put up with the intensity of the workplace or demands of a high-profile job. But in another sense, she has too many jobs. She's chauffeur, cheerleader, coach, homework monitor, and chief cook and bottle washer for her four kids and her husband, Nick.

She posts the kids' schedules on the refrigerator, listing sports commitments, clubs, after-school activities, play dates, social engagements, and doctors' appointments. But somehow, she can never keep all the schedules straight. She misses at least one essential deadline for each child each week. It's no fun knowing you've failed at your key job—being a parent—and Jessica finds herself looking forward to her evening cocktail.

Cocktail hour is her stress relief—along with the cigarette she permits herself when the kids aren't around. The solitary evening drink, with cigarettes, is really the one time of day when she can completely relax.

The situation is exacerbated by the fact that Nick doesn't get home till late at night, leaving Jessica to bear the brunt of the child-raising, disciplining, and family decision-making all by herself. Nick has always put in long hours, but a few months ago, he realized that he could get more work done on the train than being stuck in rush-hour traffic—and maybe lower his tension level, too. Unfortunately, the trains out of the city are few and far between at night, and Nick usually opts for a later one. What's more, since the family has cut back to one car, it's Jessica who must meet the train, and a few times recently, she's found herself really a bit too wobbly from exhaustion (not to mention the cocktails) to drive safely.

The Stress on All Sides

The corporate rat race has Nick so worried—half the people at his level were let go just before Christmas last year—that he works most weekends, too. Jessica tries to be supportive; their credit card debt is fairly frightening, and keeping four children fed and clothed is expensive. But it means that she and Nick barely see each other except in bed, where they are both too exhausted, worried, and agitated for the kind of intimacy that once flourished between them.

It also means that Jessica must spend her weekends attending the soccer games, track meets, and swimming competitions that occupy her children. Invariably, one of the contests will be an away game requiring a predawn wake-up. Those days, she finds herself in the kitchen, barely awake, trying to cook a hearty breakfast and get the kids ready. It's a long drive to some of those games. On arrival, she gets to watch a lot of slim, muscular children compete in sports. In fact, she told me that watching them reminds Jessica of how much weight she has put on lately.

She actually wonders why all this stress has not helped her lose weight. But the reasons are fairly obvious. While she runs a virtual catering service for the kids, she eats most of her own meals in the car or in front of the TV. By the time all her work is done, she's basically just hungry for anything that will fill her up.

A world away from the dynamic glamour of Barbara's life, Jessica is actually in exactly the same place. Her state of stress, like Barbara's, is life-shortening and life-threatening.

Where Is Your Own Stress Taking You?

In some ways, I'm sure, you identify with Barbara, with Jessica, or both. Theirs are just some of the most common stresses of everyday life. All of us face the pressure and strain of being disrupted or upset by circumstances.

But what a cost! Not only is stress itself harmful, it is also the springboard for numerous other conditions that harm us even further. It can cause us to overeat, to drink to excess, to smoke, to avoid exercise, to avoid leaving the house and connecting with others. It can make us underperform at work, renege on commitments, surrender responsibility for our relationships. In short, it can and does poison life as well as shorten it.

The Management Part

Fortunately, both Barbara and Jessica had some guidance in managing their stress. They learned how to do it without making any earthshaking changes in their lives. Barbara is still in the same high-pressure job—in fact, doing better than ever professionally. Jessica, of course, still gets the kids' meals and taxis them to their sports activities, doctors' appointments, and friends' parties. But even though the framework of both Barbara's and Jessica's lives has not been dramatically changed, each woman has a new outlook.

How did they do it?

The eleven-day "Chill" program that you find on these pages has all the components of the awareness-development and action steps that Barbara and Jessica have used in their own lives.

Quit Smoking for Life

Smoke a cigarette . . . lose eleven minutes of life.

Smoke a pack of cigarettes . . . lose three and a half hours of life.

Smoke a pack a day for a week . . . lose a day of life.

Here's a workable plan for quitting smoking. Ask your doctor for the prescriptions:

One Zyban per day for the first week

Two Zyban per day for the second week

. . . and thereafter until not needed.

Add a transdermal patch the third week if desired—and stop smoking.

This will break your habit, and you can begin to deal with the stress and other factors that caused you to smoke.

Do You Need It?

Surprisingly, neither Barbara nor Jessica was fully and consciously aware of the cost of stress in their own lives.

It's astonishing how often that's the case.

So that's the importance of awareness. Dr. Fink and Ms. Amato speak of patients who complain of headaches or stomachaches or who are angry or tired all the time, when what is really at issue is stress.

Some stressed-out people are so accustomed to feeling out of breath or anxious that they don't know any other way to feel. Ask them how they are, and they answer "Fine"—for the shortness of breath and the anxiety have simply become the norm of their lives, which are in a constant state of stress.

A vicious cycle is set in motion when patients "take a pill" for the headache or sleeplessness they feel, only to find that the cure for the first symptom has given rise to another symptom—typically in the form of stomach ulcers. Far from dealing with the real problem, people don't know what the problem is, or even that they have one.

The Wake-up Call

When Barbara came to see me, it was because she wanted to lose a few pounds. She told me she had a big conference coming up for which she wanted to look her best. And that was her main concern. Despite everything else that was going on in her life, stress was not even on her radar. Yet stress was having such a powerful effect on her that it was actually shortening her life every day.

Even when I suggested as much to her, she replied that she thrived on stress. I agreed that stress could indeed be positive. For many people, the sheer rush of adrenaline creates excitement. In fact, it's an almost addictive high that can release phenomenally creative energy. But only up to a point. In time, the activation of the stress response begins to erode creative energy, not generate it.

In my view, Barbara had come to that point and gone past it. Yes, I could help her lose her desired few pounds—even more than a few—but until she learned to manage her stress, all the related issues would sneak up on her. In all probability, she would continue to have difficulty managing her weight. As stress took its toll in terms of immunity, she would probably be sick more often, succumbing to every virus that drifted through the office. She would certainly continue to endanger her overall health and threaten her longevity.

Acute vs. Chronic Stress

One reason I emphasize awareness in the following program is because you can't manage the problem until you recognize it. But even before you begin on a stress-management program, it's important to acknowledge that there are two very different kinds of stress. Doctors have identified different categories—called *acute* and *chronic*.

What's the difference?

In the eleven-day program, I'll give you some guidelines for identifying which kind you have. But it helps to have an overview of both.

The Acute Kind

Acute stress zaps you when something has happened. Typically, that "something" is one event, occurrence, or situation that launched the stress. The dog gets sick. Your tax bill arrives, and it's twice what you expected. The roof needs to be replaced. Your child brings home a disappointing report card. Your spouse has just called to say he'll be home late. It's too hot outside. It's too cold inside. You just had a fight with your mother—again.

You react at once to these acute stresses, and the reaction is both emotional and physical. *Emotionally*, you feel the anger or resentment or unhappiness instantly. *Physically*, you find yourself undergoing such sensations as quickened pulse, rising body temperature, a feeling of dizziness, or the sudden need to sit down. You might experience tiredness, lassitude, even chest pain.

Here's a good example of acute stress: In the days after September 11, 2001, a lot of people in New York City headed for emergency rooms, believing they were having heart attacks. Despite all the symptoms and complaints, the vast majority of these people were experiencing acute stress rather than medical problems. Anger, fear, and grief unleashed by the attack on the World Trade Center had caught up with them; their stress was manifesting itself physically.

The Chronic Kind

Chronic stress, unlike acute stress, is more long term and often more insidious. It can also be far more persistent. Unlike the acute response that stems directly from a very obvious source—like a fight with your mother—chronic stress often comes from those steady worries that hover in our lives: the need to juggle bills against a salary that just isn't quite enough; the parent with Alzheimer's; the boss who treats you like dirt; the loneliness at the heart of a marriage; the looming thought of a retirement for which you're ill prepared financially and emotionally; the pressure of being overweight in a culture that worships thinness; a child in uniform, serving overseas in a dangerous place.

Worries like these don't cause you to slam down the phone, like that fight with your mother. Unlike the heart-attack symptoms that struck so many people with the acute stress after 9/11, the emotional and physical impacts of chronic stress are usually more difficult to identify. But with chronic stress, constant pressure does create symptoms over the long term. For instance, you begin to realize that there have been too many sleepless nights. You glance at your reflection in the mirror and suddenly realize how sad and stooped you look. Or, like Jessica, you start thinking earlier and earlier about the cocktail that has become your reward at the end of the day.

You might not realize you have chronic stress until you begin to wonder why you're overeating—or perhaps overdieting. But that is by no means the only signal. You may find that your palms are sweaty, you can't concentrate, you're aware of frequent and inexplicable mood swings. Or you feel as if your energy is being steadily sapped, dripping away drop by drop, day after day. You're tied up in knots, but you're afraid that if the string is pulled, you'll unravel altogether. Emotionally and physically, this is what chronic stress feels like.

Dealing with Both Kinds

There are ways to manage acute or chronic stress. Sometimes, it's possible to eliminate or adjust the cause of the acute stress. In certain cases, it can be waited out. If your spouse is late getting home from work, your stress and all its physical symptoms may disappear soon after he arrives.

With acute stress, you may begin to feel relief as soon as you take some sort of action that deflates the cause. The action reminds you that you do have control. Your feeling of stress is replaced by a sense that you're able to handle the situation, a feeling of accomplishment. You take the sick dog to the vet, or you get a tutor to help your academically challenged child, and your stress dissipates—along with the breathlessness or sleeplessness or other physical symptom.

When the stress is chronic, however, you will probably find it harder to identify the source and deal with the causes. In fact, rooting out the source of chronic stress often requires life-changing actions. If being overweight is a source of chronic stress, it won't be enough to lose weight today—like Barbara taking off a few pounds. Instead, you will need to change your entire relationship with food so that the chronic nature of your overweight ends once and for all.

As for the boss who contributes to chronic stress by treating you badly, your plan of action requires some decision-making. You might simply decide that you will put up with the bad treatment because you're so well paid—it's worth it! (Surprising as it may seem, even with a decision like that, your stress diminishes.) The other thing you can say to yourself is that the *stress is part of the job itself*; that is, it's just part of the daily task of showing up and doing the work—not something that you can change by trying to alter your boss's behavior. So if you stick with the job, you'll have to accept that you need to deal with this aspect of it.

On the other hand, depending on the nature of your boss's bad treatment of you, you might have to work out a solution through your Human Resources department or by bringing a lawsuit. Or you might choose to quit your job: that would inevitably lead to the stress of looking for another job, but it is still a highly effective way to end the chronic stress of working for someone whose treatment of you is poisoning your life. Obviously, many of these actions cannot be taken immediately without thoughtful preparation, and that's where counseling can come in handy.

Then, too, there are some sources of chronic stress that are simply outside our control. There is no cure for Alzheimer's. There is no way to avoid mandated retirement. You cannot order your child in the armed forces to come home and live a safe life near you; you can only watch the news and hope. These are stress sources you simply cannot reach, much less control. Yet *there are ways,* using the awareness and action in the eleven-day program, *by which you can chill the negative feelings.* Attitude, and actions, can determine your outlook and help prevent chronic stress from harming your health.

But it all begins with awareness.

CHILL

THE ELEVEN-DAY PROGRAM

DAYS 1–4: THE AWARENESS DAYS

If you're going to be able to manage your stress, you must first get to know it. What is its source? What triggers it? How does it affect you? How big is it—that is, how powerful a role does it play in your life?

In the first four days of the eleven-day program, you will identify your stress, get a picture of it, inventory the factors that drive it, and understand what it's doing to you. In a very real sense, I'm asking you to play detective over the next four days, to objectively investigate the stress in your life.

Day 1: Discover where your stress is.

Everyone has stress. Where's yours?

Today you're going to find out, using two questionnaires that will help you discover it and even measure it.

What follows is a copyrighted test created and distributed by BlueCross BlueShield to keep the public informed about health care. The test consists of a list of life events, each of which has been assigned a point value. *Go down the list of events one at a time, and find the events that have applied to you over the course of the last year—just one year. Then add up your points.*

Life Event	Points
Death of spouse	100
Divorce	73
Marital separation	65
Jail term	63
Death of close family member	63
Personal injury or illness	53
Marriage	50
Fired at work	47
Marital reconciliation	45
Retirement	45
Change in health of family member	44
Pregnancy	40
Sex difficulties	39
Gain of new family member	39
Business readjustment	39
Change in financial state	38
Death of close friend	37
Change to different line of work	36
Change in number of arguments with spouse	35
Mortgage over $10,000	31
Foreclosure of mortgage or loan	30
Change in responsibilities at work	29
Son or daughter leaving home	29

Life Event	Points
Trouble with in-laws	29
Outstanding personal achievement	26
Spouse begins or leaves a job	26
Begin or end school	25
Change in living conditions	25
Change in personal habits	24
Trouble with boss	23
Change in work hours or conditions	20
Change in residence	20
Change in schools	20
Change in church activities	19
Change in recreation	19
Change in social activities	18
Mortgage or loan less than $10,000	17
Change in sleeping habits	16
Change in number of family get-togethers	15
Change in eating habits	13
Vacation	13
Christmas (December-January holiday season)	12
Minor violations of the law	11
	TOTAL: _____

How did you score? If your list puts you below 150 points, you have approximately a one-in-three chance of confronting a worsening health situation in the next two years.

If you scored between 150 and 300, you have a 50-50 chance of a serious and adverse health change in the next two years.

If you scored *higher than 300*, you face a *90 percent likelihood of a change for the worse* in your health within the next two years.

As this evaluation makes abundantly clear, the higher the number of stress factors (particularly high-point factors), the more negative the impact on your health and longevity.

When Do *You* Feel Most Stressed?

The second questionnaire (on the next page) helps you size up your stress—literally. But instead of listing specific events like the previous test, the next evaluation refers to general situations. In order for the test to give you a fair reading of stress factors in your life, you will need to answer with complete honesty.

The column on the left describes ten common situations in which you might find yourself. For each situation, determine the extent to which the situation would stress you out. Assess your stress level on a scale of 1 to 5, where 5 is very stressed and 1 is not at all stressed. Check the appropriate column. If the situation simply doesn't apply to you, just put a check mark in the column headed "Not applicable."

I feel stressed when . . .						
		Very				**Not at all**	**Not applicable**
		5	4	3	2	1	0
1	I'm away from my family						
2	I'm at a party						
3	I'm at work						
4	I have to deal with conflict						
5	I have to make a decision						
6	someone I love is ill						
7	I have to change an appointment						
8	I have to compete at work or play						
9	I am being observed at play						
10	I am being observed at work						
	Totals						
	OVERALL TOTAL: _____						

Add up your stress values by column, then compute your total number of points. This is your stress score. Here's how your stress measures up:

If you scored . . .	Then you are . . .
41–50	Very stressed
31–40	Moderately stressed
21–30	Mildly stressed
20 or below	Very calm

The questionnaire tells you more than how stressed you are, however. It helps you identify the kinds of events, situations, or experiences that create an environment where you feel the most stress.

Take another look at the ten situations, particularly the ones in which you scored 5, 4, or even 3. How do these situations get to you?

Maybe you're a teacher who becomes utterly flustered when a supervisor or the principal drops into the classroom to "observe." Are you worried he or she will find you doing something wrong? Are you stressed out from concerns about your own level of competence?

Or perhaps you're someone who simply cannot make up your mind when you're looking at a restaurant menu. You get stressed at the need to decide on one dish out of all the choices on the menu. Are you afraid your dinner companions will in some way judge your choice—and find you wanting as a result? What is it about the need to make a decision that really bothers you? You may be afraid to make the wrong choice. But you know what? It's okay, we all do, it's part of the journey.

I encourage you—for the purpose of greater awareness—to again think hard about what precisely stresses you out, particularly in the situations in which you scored a 5 or 4. Try to evaluate the contributing factors as honestly as you can. Then boil it all down to the simplest, shortest description, as follows:

The source of my stress is _____.

With the results of these two questionnaires in hand, you now have a better idea of what you're up against. You know the potential danger of your stress, you've taken its measure, and given it a name.

Results of Day 1: *You've found your sources of stress.*

Day 2: Is it chronic or acute?

How do you differentiate between chronic and acute stress?

One way is to start with a simple question. *Ask yourself whether the source of your stress can be changed. If so, that is acute stress.*

The next thing to figure out is how that source of stress can end. If you're racing to meet a deadline, for instance, you know that the acute stress will end as soon as you've completed the job or assignment and met that deadline. Or suppose you're training for a bicycle trip and you're feeling a lot of stress because you don't know whether it's too tough for you. Or let's say there's a new hire who's clearly gunning for your job, making every day in the office more stressful. These all are events, situations, or experiences that can in some way be altered or that can disappear altogether.

In some cases, it may just be a question of time before the stress passes. In other cases (as in the case of the bike ride), you can find ways to simply take the pressure off—by not doing the bike ride or, if it's too tough, just dropping out and cycling back to the start. In still other cases, the event or situation or experience will take place and then be over. For instance, if the new hire turns out to be incompetent and gets fired, your job will no longer feel threatened, and that particular acute stress will go away.

Acute stresses, in short, *are solvable: the source of the stress can be made to go away, and the stress will go away too.*

And it is important to know that.

With chronic stress, as I've pointed out, *the source of stress may be beyond your control.* In a situation where you have a parent with Alzheimer's, the stress will not go away until the parent's death. Both the fact of your parent's disease and the stress that it causes are things you must live with—*but you can change the way you deal with it*.

But that's only one scenario. **Some sources of chronic stress can be changed**. Suppose you've been married for twenty years, and for nineteen years, you've been miserable. Or perhaps you go to work every day for a boss you hate. You can end your marriage; you could quit your job. In the meantime, however, if you choose to do neither, you're living with chronic stress that you feel like you can't change. **With chronic stresses like these, the only solution is to learn how to change the way you deal with the cause of stress.**

That is why understanding the nature of your stress—chronic or acute, or both—is so important. So, today, try to evaluate carefully and honestly whether the stress you feel comes from a source that can be changed or not. This evaluation will form the basis of your ability to manage your stress, either by changing the source of stress (if it can be changed) or learning to live with it (if it can't).

To make the evaluation, just ask yourself:

"Can the source of my stress be eliminated by the passage of time and the normal turn of events, by me, or by someone else?"

If the answer is yes, your stress is solvable. If the answer is no, you will have to learn to live with it or change the way you deal with it.

Results of Day 2: *You've evaluated your stress and you understand its nature.*

Day 3: Complete a "stress trigger" inventory.

There's a difference between the *source* of your stress and things that *trigger* the feeling of stress.

When you identify the source, you have figured out the reason you feel stress. But when you're looking for stress triggers, you need to identify the specific incidents or occurrences that precipitate a stress reaction.

For example, for one of my patients, Susan, the source of stress was her weight. She had fought the battle of the bulge all her life, losing and then regaining weight in the classic scenario of the perpetual dieter. Being overweight was a solvable chronic stress that affected every aspect of her life.

And then she discovered that supermarket shopping was one of her triggers. Whenever she had to shop, Susan felt momentarily paralyzed into a state of inaction. But what triggered this reaction? After all, it was her weight that was stressing her out—not the orderly, well-stocked supermarket where she had been a customer for years. And it wasn't that she necessarily feared bingeing, either. Even if she had a list of innocuous supplies—like coffee, bottled water, skim milk, paper towels, laundry detergent—she still felt daunted by the prospect of visiting the supermarket.

The more Susan probed, the clearer the issue became. She realized there was one male supermarket clerk who invariably looked her up and down as she was paying for her purchases. This would happen whether or not she was in the clerk's checkout line. She just "knew" it was because she was so overweight. In her mind, the guy looking at her was seeing a fat woman—undesirable, unappealing, unacceptable, an outcast. No wonder she could barely put one foot in front of the other when she had to head for the supermarket.

For Susan, it was *the experience of going* to the supermarket that *triggered her stress* reaction, even though the source of her stress was the pressure of being overweight.

To inventory your stress triggers, go back to the questionnaires of Day 1. *For both the life-event list and the ten situations, put a star next to each statement or description you recognize as a trigger.*

When you've done that, *look over the list.* These are your personal triggers. Whenever you encounter these situations, you can expect your stress level to soar. But by recognizing those triggers and being ready for them, you can get set to manage stress.

Results of Day 3: *You understand what triggers your stress reactions.*

Day 4: *Get in touch with the feelings that come from the stress you have.*

Some people can go days, weeks, or even months without giving much thought to how they're feeling. We get used to saying things that seem to express emotions but really don't—like "I'm really exhausted," "It's a nice day," or "This is frustrating."

There's a big difference between these kinds of expressions and a real articulation of feelings. When I speak of the major classifications of feelings, I am looking for words like **sadness, gladness, anger, frustration, fear, guilt, or excitement.**

To deal with your stress, you need to be aware of feelings. And then you need to take the next step, doing what psychologists always advocate—that is, *allow yourself to feel the feelings.*

That may sound simple, but when you're not fully aware of your feelings, they need to be deciphered. And until they are—until you can feel the feelings—your stress level builds and builds.

Let's take one example from the workplace. Suppose you're expected to give a presentation to the head of your division in just three hours. Like a lot of people in that situation, you know that a lot is riding on your performance. Just three hours to prepare, with the danger that your whole career is on the line. Of course there's pressure, and it's making you a little short of breath.

Another example, this one on the home front. Suppose, today, you just don't want to read or hear about the local crimes and disasters or the national crises that are so disturbing. So you try to avoid reading the front page of the newspaper. But by accident, you catch a bit of the evening news on television. Before you can grab the remote and channel-surf away from the headlines, you already have a headache. You feel all too helpless in the face of war, terrorism, and natural disasters, and you're sure it's not good for your blood pressure to know what's going on in the world.

Or take a typical commute to and from work. For many people, it means an hour or more of anger and frustration. Driving seems to have become a way to prove something; everyone is out to gain advantage, and courtesy is unknown. Or you're riding a train or bus that's overcrowded, often late, and filled with tense people. The result: You get home from work and reach for a stiff drink to help compensate for the rotten time you've just had.

Out of breath. Suffering from headache. Alcohol-dependent. All are symptoms of stress. But these symptoms mask underlying feelings. The problem is, people defer the expression of those feelings. But *unless they're acknowledged, they're likely to erupt in dangerous and destructive ways.*

If you're going to be able to cope with your stress, you'll need to go beneath the symptoms to get in touch with the underlying emotions or feelings.

To do that, accept the physical symptoms as signals of stress.

Understand that these are clues. They provide evidence about the stress that's getting in the way of your functioning. Pursue these clues, and they'll tell you not just what you're feeling but also what you're thinking when stress gets in the way of your life.

To help you get a clearer understanding of your own feelings, start by drawing up a chart with four columns, like this:

The Symptom	Emotions or Feelings	The Situation	The Thought

In the first column, note the physical symptom, such as racing pulse, headache, clenched teeth, or the need for a drink to help you calm down.

In the second column, note your underlying feelings. What were you feeling when your pulse was racing? Can you identify how you felt a few moments before your head started pounding? When you got home from your commute and immediately poured yourself a glass of wine, what was the feeling behind that impulse? Go find that feeling again. Was it sadness? Anger? Frustration? Guilt? Fear? A happy excitement?

These are not the only clues.

Have you ever found yourself suddenly crying for no reason that you can fathom? You're in the grip of a profound **sadness**.

Perhaps you had a headache for days; it wouldn't go away. Now you see that the emotion connected with that symptom is **fear**.

Or maybe three different coworkers at the office have remarked that you seem annoyed about something. You admit it: You're **angry**.

In each of these instances, you may have to do some real

searching before you learn about the feeling that lies behind the symptom.

And then there are feelings that are more difficult to admit. Dr. Fink gives this example: Let's say you have a young daughter and you promised you'd come to her chorus recital. It turns out that the time of her recital is in conflict with a make-or-break meeting at the office. So you feel **guilty** about missing the recital. But at another level, there may be a feeling that's much more difficult to admit—let's say you're actually **glad** you don't have to go to the recital. You're looking forward to the important business meeting with feelings of **excitement**. Thanks to these feelings of **happiness**, your **guilt** vis-à-vis your daughter feels like a ten-ton truck you're wearing around your neck.

In a situation like this, it's no wonder that you might try to censor some of those feelings by rating them "unacceptable." But you can't change those feelings or deny them. And if you try, you'll end up without any idea whether you really feel a certain way or whether you just know you're supposed to feel a certain way.

The answer? Let yourself feel these feelings, Dr. Fink says—and that means without judging whether they're negative or positive. Don't think. Don't analyze. Just experience the emotion. Then name it, and write it down in column two.

In *column three, set down the situation that has stimulated your uncomfortable emotion.* Something is getting in the way of your life. That could be the reason why you're having headaches, or barking at coworkers, or finding yourself in tears.

Can you identify the situation that brought on this reaction? What kicked off the headache? Not fear—that is the feeling. *But what situation caused the fear?* What's going on at home or in the office that is shortening your fuse with coworkers? What on earth made the tears well up in your eyes—something that never happens? Find what precipitated the emotion that has you in its power. Write it down.

Now turn to the fourth column and try to evaluate the thought associated with the emotion. For instance, you might figure out that your annoyance level at the office shot up when you received a mediocre performance review. You're quite simply afraid for your job, and it has made you emotionally low. I'm incompetent, you've been thinking to yourself. There's no way I can do this job.

Or perhaps you determine that your headache springs from a fear that was sparked by a fight you had with your spouse. Maybe what's really bothering you is not that particular fight, but the fact that it duplicates the kind of fights that you've been having for years. The fear you're feeling arises from concern that there's a serious gulf you may not be able to bridge: What will this mean? What if the marriage is over? What happens to my life?

Yes, some of these thoughts may be exaggerations, half-truths, or pure imaginings. That doesn't matter for the moment. The important thing is to write down what you're thinking.

Finally, take a look at what you've written. Are your true feelings and thoughts distasteful to you? Do you feel guilty about feeling what you feel? Put the guilt or distaste aside, and let yourself, as Ms. Amato advises, "feel the feelings." They are real, and they belong to you. You're allowed to feel them, and you need to feel them if you are to manage the stress they're producing.

It may be hard to get used to the idea that you can't manage stress by dismissing your feelings or not allowing yourself to admit them. But all the studies of stress management show that if you feel guilty about your feelings, and try to deny them, your stress just gets worse. Reach down to touch your feelings now so that they don't surface later to harm you more harshly.

Results of Day 4: *You have allowed yourself to feel what's stressing you out.*

DAYS 5–11: THE ACTION DAYS

By now, you have a good idea of where your stress comes from, what it looks like, what it feels like, and what it's doing to your life. It's time now to take action to deal with it.

Understand that this won't be an easy ride. Backsliding is almost inevitable. In fact, just about everybody backslides; we go back to the behavior we know because it's comfortable—and because it's ours. There's even a psychological term for it: egosyntonic—having our ego in synch with our behavior.

When you are in a pattern of egosyntonic behavior, it's likely that you're doing a lot of things that make you feel good simply because they're familiar. The well-tried patterns always seem the most acceptable.

But what if those patterns are contributing to stress rather than helping you manage it? In the next seven days, you're going to start doing some unfamiliar things. That means you have to ***dare to change the things you think you can't change***. In doing so, you will learn to both confront and manage your stress.

Day 5: Learn not to panic.

ca·tas·tro·phe (kə-tas trə-fē) noun

1. A great, often sudden calamity. A disaster.
2. A complete failure; a fiasco.
3. A cataclysm.

Does your situation qualify for this dictionary definition of a catastrophe? Does it really feel like the end of the world? What's actually going on? Even if a situation seems like a catastrophe, isn't there a way you can gain a measure of control over it?

In the summer of 2004, Dawn, a former patient of mine, and her husband, Robert, retired and relocated to Florida's east coast. They moved into their dream house. They had saved for this house for nearly fifty years, and it took five years to design and build.

Robert and Dawn spent two happy months in their new home. Then Hurricane Frances came barreling up the coast. The couple was evacuated to a shelter. During their absence, the hurricane took down a tree that crashed through the roof of the house. Torrents of rain flooded the first floor, ruining furniture, carpets, and many of their dearest possessions. When they returned from the shelter and saw what had become of their retirement dream, Dawn and Robert both wept.

Then Dawn said to Robert: "We're alive."

They got a pump, grabbed a broom, and went to work. Three weeks later, with the power turned on again, with insurance adjusters and federal emergency-management officials offering them hope, and with things feeling like they just might get better, Hurricane Jeanne arrived. Another evacuation, and when Robert and Dawn again returned to their half-repaired home, they found more damage and destruction. For the second time in a month, they wept over the loss of a dream. And for the second time in a month, they picked up their tools and went to work to recover what they could and rebuild their home and their lives. "This time," quipped Dawn, "we know how to do it."

There is always something you know how to do other than panicking, other than letting the situation—any situation—become a disaster in your own mind. **Stress can make every situation seem like a catastrophe**. By doing the something you can do, you both lessen the "catastrophe" and reduce your stress.

It's a way of taking charge. Control anything at all that you can control—even if it's just a broom—and you feel greater mastery over the situation as a whole. Dawn and Robert could not fight the hurricanes or undo its damage, but they could pump the water out of their living room, sweep up the mess, and get the reconstruction process underway.

Note, neither of them was an expert at this sort of disaster response. Neither Robert nor Dawn knew much about building repair. And there were many contingencies that they could *not* control—the lack of electrical power, for instance. But by doing what they could, they got out of the mode of thinking "this is a complete catastrophe." They put their situation in perspective and punctured their own panic.

That is what you are going to learn to do today. Start with a sheet of paper that gives you plenty of room to write. Then make three columns, like this:

Catastrophe	Not Really	What I Can Do

In the first column, write down everything about your situation that makes you regard it as a catastrophe. For example, an expected promotion didn't come through. If you dwell on that event, you might find yourself thinking that your days with the company are numbered. Take it further (with catastrophic thinking) and you could start to believe that you'll never have another chance in your chosen career. Your prospects throughout the industry are dim. That panic, in turn, will get you thinking about your ability to keep making payments on your house, maintain your standard of living, enjoy the future you've planned.

Now look at what you've written. To fill in the second column, change your perspective. How real was your expectation of the promotion? Could it have been more fantasy than probability? How many candidates qualified for this promotion, and where—honestly—did you rank among them? Maybe you shouldn't have expected the promotion after all.

Or maybe not getting the promotion can serve as a career signal. In the "Not Really" column, you might find yourself writing, "Maybe it's a good thing." And, indeed, maybe there's reason to be grateful for this early warning sign. Perhaps it's a hint that you should look elsewhere for a job, or retrain, or find some new challenges at the place where you're now employed. What seemed a catastrophe—seen one way—can be seen as a useful wake-up call when you start to fill in the "Not Really" column.

With changed perspective, you have an opportunity to see the "disaster" in another light. ***It's not a catastrophe anymore. It's a situation that affects you.*** But you play a part in that situation, and there are actions you can take.

In column three, write down the things that you can do about the situation. What is within your power?

For example, if you didn't get the promotion you expected, you can talk to your supervisor to find out why you were passed over. That's just one alternative. Or what about seeking a transfer? Looking for a job outside the firm? Or perhaps taking classes and getting credentials for some other line of work? Alternatively, you could buckle down, redouble your efforts, and aim to show that you deserve the next promotion.

Keep writing. In that third column, list every action you can possibly do. Then look at all the possibilities. That's a pretty full agenda for dealing with what seemed to be a full-blown catastrophe just a little while ago.

By finding things that you can do, you end your sense of helplessness, reduce "catastrophe" to a manageable situation, and establish yourself as the one who is going to do the managing.

Results of Day 5: *You have punctured the panic, taken control, and empowered yourself.*

A Meditation Medley

Although comedians may scoff at people who meditate—with jokes about New Age bliss, bells, and mantras—it's the meditators who will have the last laugh. Here's just some of what the latest science has proven about this most ancient of practices.

- Statistics show that meditation extends life.
- Laboratory studies demonstrate that meditation boosts the immune system.
- Brain scans reveal that meditation may be "rewiring" the brain to reduce stress and reshaping it to respond to crises without a spike in blood pressure.
- Medical research has found that meditation may help prevent, slow, or control chronic pain from such diseases as heart disease, AIDS, cancer, or infertility.
- Psychiatric research recommends meditation to restore balance in people suffering from depression, hyperactivity, and attention deficit disorder (ADD).
- Meditation has been shown to reverse plaque buildup in the arteries of some patients and to slow prostate cancer in others.
- Psoriasis patients who meditated enjoyed skin clearing four times faster than nonmeditators.
- A combination of meditation and guided imagery raised the level of the immune cells known to combat breast tumors in some women.
- Meditation can significantly reduce blood pressure.
- Meditators have been shown to use less oxygen, lower their heart rates, and increase the brain waves that appear right before sleep during meditation, achieving a calm, happy state.

Day 6: Relax.

As your actions start to win out over catastrophic thinking, you'll feel the panic diminish. Now you can prepare to take care of yourself.

Taking care of yourself is perhaps the most effective antidote to stress. Today, you begin to physically combat your stress by being good to yourself.

It starts with relaxing. You have to get into a physically relaxed state to relieve the tension or strain that is the manifestation of your stress.

There are numerous relaxation techniques, but I recommend the following four as a great starting point. To get the most out of these, I suggest that you do them all at least three times during the day.

1. *Breathe deeply.* Shallow breathing is a characteristic of panic, so begin by slowly taking a deep breath. Expand your whole diaphragm, the area below your chest. Make sure you don't lift your shoulders or tense your neck. Just let your stomach rise and fall. With each expansion of your abdomen, you effortlessly take air into your lungs. Then exhale like a balloon deflating—but slowly.

2. *Meditate.* I'm only going to ask that you meditate for a minute. Turn off all phones, TVs, radios, stereos, and other sounds. Sit comfortably. Although some people hum or repeat a phrase (mantra) in meditation, you don't need to do that. The goal is to empty your mind, and the easiest way to do that is by focusing on your breath. As you breathe deeply, in and out, think about . . . nothing! If you find your mind drifting to specific problems—your plans, schedule, or obligations— label that "thinking." Go back to focusing on your breath.

3. *Stretch.* Stretching gets the blood flowing and helps you maximize the range of motion of your joints, keeping your body flexible. It makes you feel good, and nothing is better for deterring stress. Stretch upward, sideward, downward. Everybody knows basic fitness stretches that can be done anywhere, at any time.

4. *Imagine.* Close your eyes, take a few measured breaths, and transport yourself to someplace you love. Maybe it's a picture you yourself paint of fantasy surroundings, or perhaps you want to bring into your mind the image of a place you know well. Focus on the details: colors, textures, sounds, smells. If it's a beach, try to feel the sand between your toes. If it's the woods, listen for the sounds of birds singing. Stay in this beautiful place for a few minutes—an excellent way to relieve tension and relax the body.

Results of Day 6: *You have learned relaxation techniques to overcome stress.*

Give Yourself a Day Off

One great way to embrace pleasure is to be pampered. Let somebody else take care of you for a day! That's what spas are all about. They offer so many of the things that make us feel better and that we've talked about as antidotes to stress: massage, exercise, creative activities, meditation, nutrition, and more.

I'm a great believer in the effectiveness of spas and routinely prescribe spa treatment for my New York City–based patients. Many of them are not even aware of all the "little" stresses they undergo each day as residents of the world's most exciting city—waiting for a bus or hailing a taxi, dodging bicycle messengers, living with the noise of traffic and construction and honking horns. I estimate that seven out of ten of my patients suffer chronic neck and back muscle tension aches and aren't even aware that they're tense because the tension is so universal and so routine. Spas, in short, cure these patients of ills they didn't know they had.

Of course, you can also fly off to a spa resort. But even if you just take off one day to go to a spa, you'll get a good break from routine. It's a way to take yourself out of your usual environment and enter a place where people are dedicated to taking care of you. You're there for one reason—to feel good—and with staff dancing attendance upon you, you can easily let go of all the things that may be stressing you out.

Day 7: Use positive self-talk.

You talk to yourself all the time. We all do. Today, you're going to make sure that everything you say to yourself is positive.

During a normal day, there are many opportunities to give yourself a positive self-talk. But let's take one situation as an example.

You've been invited to a party. You walk in alone. Glancing around the room, you quickly realize that you don't know anyone there. Everywhere around you, groups of people are chatting. It will be hard to break in. You feel self-conscious, suddenly aware that you're wearing the wrong outfit, or feeling like you don't belong, or worried that you have nothing interesting to say.

This is the moment for positive self-talk. *Say to yourself: "I can do this. I belong here as much as anyone else in the room. I have something to offer these people. I am valuable in my own right."*

Even when you're alone, there are likely to be times throughout the day when you need to give yourself a positive self-talk. Let's say you go to lunch intending to have a salad and nothing more. But at the end of the meal, you can't resist a special dessert. What do you say afterward? One scenario is that you beat yourself up: *"I blew it, I can't believe I ate the dessert, I'll never lose weight."*

But that just increases your stress. Instead, try telling yourself: *"Okay, I'm disappointed, but not being perfect is part of the process or journey, and here's what I can do about it: I can take charge, accept that I've done it, and move on with the journey."*

Or suppose you have a big presentation tomorrow. If you remind yourself that this presentation is terribly important and you have always been nervous about public speaking, your stress level is likely to soar. That's because you're emphasizing the fear factors, the negatives. Instead, manage stress by telling yourself the positives over and over: "*I know this material; nobody knows it better.* It's natural to feel nervous, and it's okay to feel nervous; the nervousness is energy I can use. I have carefully organized this presentation. I have rehearsed it. I can do this well. I'll be fine."

Positive self-talk affirms your own worth. It reminds you about your own competence. As you learned on Day 5 (how not to panic), there is always another perspective—and positive self-talk is a powerful way to remind yourself of that other way of looking at things.

Make this internal dialogue personal, supportive, and realistic. Speak to yourself in the present tense and talk in terms of achievable, believable goals.

Just for practice—to get used to this positive-talk exercise— here are five affirmations I'd like you to repeat to yourself at least three times during the day:

1. My special expertise is _____.
2. I can lead a healthy life.
3. I like the way I look; my best feature is _____.
4. If I fall apart, I know it's not forever, and I know how to put myself together again.
5. I have what it takes; I believe in me. I'm well prepared.

Results of Day 7: *With positive self-talk, you have told yourself you're fine—and you believe it.*

Day 8: Think positive.

We all know people who live in the land of **but**. No matter how sensational the event or experience, "they're careful to note the downside," says Ms. Amato. They vacation for three weeks in Hawaii, but their main impression is that the flowers were overwhelming. They go to lunch at a fancy restaurant, *but they tell* you that it felt second-rate because there was iceberg lettuce in the salad. They get tickets to a hit Broadway show, *but* they talk mostly about how costly the drinks were at intermission.

Now, it's interesting to note that all these observations may be absolutely true and correct. Hawaii's blooms are extravagant. First-class restaurants sometimes serve iceberg lettuce. A drink in a Broadway theater can cost an arm and a leg. The question is, which was the more valuable—the positive aspect of the experience or the negative? To people living in the land of *but*, it is the minuscule negative that dominates the experience, rather than the acres of pleasure they could have enjoyed.

This kind of negative thinking—this particular view of the world—brings on the stress that loses jobs, ruins relationships, and makes people angry, overweight, and unhappy. If you have a tendency to think that way, this day will be very important. It doesn't take much to shift the emphasis from negative to positive thinking—and once you do it, you'll begin to feel the rewards quickly.

Choose a single incident or experience from the day—at home, in the office, while shopping, while visiting with friends. Draw up a two-column list, as follows:

Negative	Positive

In the left-hand column, write down all the negative things you can think of about this incident or experience. In the right-hand column, write down all the positive things that come to mind.

For example, suppose you went shopping with a friend. The negatives might be: It was hard to find a parking space close to the shops; your friend bought a gorgeous dress that you couldn't possibly have fit into; the new bag you admired was way too expensive; all you ended up with were a bunch of staple items you needed for the house.

Positives? You spent time with someone you care about; she found a dress she loves—which made her happy; you showed admirable restraint in not buying a bag you couldn't afford; you stocked up on needed supplies. You could even add that since you had to park so far from the shops, you got some exercise with a brisk walk to and from the car.

Once you have filled in both columns, take your pen and X out each of the negatives, one by one. Concentrate on the positives only.

Results of Day 8: *You have accentuated the positive and eliminated the negative.*

Day 9: Embrace pleasure.

If you want to keep stress permanently under control, you need to recognize the rewards in your life and allow yourself to enjoy them. Feed your physical appetites with rich experiences. For some people, that might mean the luxury of a massage or a visit to the spa. For others, it's a leisurely meal, or sex, or a long, hot bath.

Taking care of yourself means embracing pleasure. *Going toward pleasure takes you away from stress* and all its tensions and physical effects. So today, I want you to do at least one very sensually enriching thing. If it's a massage you want, make an appointment. Have sex. Dine at a restaurant where the food is great and the service is wonderful. Pamper yourself with a manicure or pedicure. Best of all would be for you to do all of these things—if all appeal to you. But if that's impossible, just feed at least one physical appetite and enjoy at least one sensual pleasure.

This is a sound medical prescription, and here's why. ***Whereas stress depletes the body's energy and erodes your health, physical and sensual pleasure make measurable contributions to a sense of well-being.*** The pleasure center of your brain prompts the release of endorphins, the neurotransmitters that lead to feelings of happiness. In other words, the emotional response has a powerful and measurable physical component. With the stimulation of hormones that affect pleasure, you also balance your appetite, increase the sex drive, and strengthen the immune response. Pleasure, in short, is good for your health.

A massage, or even a manicure or pedicure, can have a similar impact; it's all about you, about taking care of you, about making you feel good.

Sex and Longevity

A study reported in the *British Medical Journal* found that men who have sex twice a week or more had half the risk of death of those who had sex less frequently than once a month.

Sex is, of course, *a great stress reliever as well*—and you don't have to leave home or make a reservation or pay a lot of money to enjoy its benefits. Sexual activity triggers hormonal and metabolic actions that restore tissue, pump oxygen around the body, enhance circulation, even help the flow of nutrients to the skin. Because it's exercise as well, sex is good for your blood pressure, muscles, and heart.

Whichever sensual pleasure you embrace will help replace your stress. Though the substitution of pleasure may seem temporary, you make extraordinary gains whenever you can break the hold of stress on your life.

Results of Day 9: *You have chased away stress with sensual pleasure.*

Day 10: Feed your soul.

Today you will feed your aesthetic appetites.

What does your soul crave? Perhaps you like music, art, or literature. But in the category of "aesthetic," I like to include every kind of amusement, pastime, and entertainment. For some, it's a movie or ball game. For others, the aesthetic appetites are fed by taking a quiet walk in the woods or going to a park where you can watch a bird in flight.

Any aesthetic pleasure sends signals to your brain that, like sensual pleasures, break the stress pattern. So today, all you have to do is choose. Here are just a few possibilities:

- Read any book that you enjoy.
- Go to a play or concert—even by yourself. (You don't need a companion when you're taking in aesthetic pleasure.)
- Wander through a museum or art gallery—and really see what you're looking at.
- Go catch a movie that you've wanted to see—for the pure joy of entertainment.

If you're not sure what gives you aesthetic pleasure, today is the day to find out. What is it that takes you out of your busy life to a different place in your brain? What is it that feeds your soul?

Results of Day 10: *You have broken the hold stress has on you by seeking an experience of aesthetic pleasure.*

Day 11: Create something!

Nothing is more life-affirming—and therefore more stress-negating—than the sense of accomplishment you feel when you create something that's completely new.

The very process of creating is both a distraction from stress and a rejection of it. When you make something, you are in control. As soon as you bring something new into being, you'll feel much more power over your environment and your life than previously. The competence you exhibit is a repudiation of the lack of control that stress gives you. And the accomplishment of having created something is a boost to self-esteem.

The possibilities are limitless, and what you choose to create will depend on what you really enjoy doing. But just to start your planning for this day, here are some possibilities:

- Start to knit a sweater.
- Plan a gourmet meal.
- Dig a garden.
- Paint a picture.
- Clean your closets.
- Build a birdhouse.
- Rearrange your desk.
- Take photographs.

In other words, do anything that you can accomplish from start to finish. Creation nullifies stress. Where stress destroys, creation builds. Where stress frustrates, accomplishment elates. Where stress drags you down, creation lifts you up and sets you free.

Results of Day 11: *You are managing your stress.*

Get Up, Get Out, Get Moving

Awareness			
DAY 1	**DAY 2**	**DAY 3**	**DAY 4**
Determine what shape you are in.	What do you want exercise to do for you?	What kind of exercise do you prefer?	Make a calendar of your exercise commitment.

Action						
DAY 5	**DAY 6**	**DAY 7**	**DAY 8**	**DAY 9**	**DAY 10**	**DAY 11**
Do push-ups to help develop upper-body strength.	Do dips to further develop upper-body strength.	Practice squats to develop lower-body strength.	Learn how to do side lunges for lower-body strength.	Do the plank for core-body strength.	Practice opposite arm and leg extensions.	Learn the power punch.

Chapter 3

GET UP, GET OUT, GET MOVING

These days, you can barely pick up a newspaper or magazine without seeing a headline about yet another study identifying yet another benefit of exercise.

It's not fiction. Exercise literally saves your life, lengthens your years, injects you with more energy, and helps every organ in your entire body work better. Here are eleven things that exercise has been proven to do for you:

1. Reduce your risk of premature death
2. Reduce your risk of heart disease
3. Reduce high blood pressure or the risk of developing it
4. Reduce high cholesterol or the risk of developing it
5. Reduce the risk of colon cancer and breast cancer
6. Reduce the risk of diabetes
7. Reduce or maintain body weight or body fat
8. Build and maintain healthy muscles, bones, and joints
9. Reduce depression and anxiety
10. Improve psychological well-being and strengthen your immune system.
11. Enhance your performance at work, at play, and in

sports

Stopping the Clock on Aging

Scientists confirm that the human body pretty much "finishes" at around age thirty. After that, preserving strength and cardiovascular fitness is up to the individual. The good news is that recent research suggests that *we can preserve strength and fitness—stopping the aging clock where it is or even turning it back—through a program of regular exercise.* Studies show that men between the ages of thirty-five and seventy-four who exercise regularly have a far greater life expectancy than their counterparts who do not exercise.

In fact, the exercisers can look forward to living an hour or two longer for every hour of exercise they do. Organ functioning, flexibility, muscle strength, metabolic rate, endurance, and stamina all improve dramatically with exercise. These are exactly the same characteristics of people who live the longest, healthiest lives. Lack of exercise, by contrast, accounts for about 50 percent of the physical decline that occurs between the ages of thirty and seventy.

Keeping Your Heart in Good Shape

As for the benefits of exercise for heart health, they are almost incalculable. In fact, medical experts agree that *most cardiovascular disease*, the number-one cause of premature death, *is self-inflicted.*

There are 80,000 miles of blood vessels in the body—a vast and complex system. Over time, such preventable things as stress, smoking, alcohol or drug abuse, an unhealthy relationship with food, high cholesterol, and high blood pressure all can clog up the system and bring it to a halt. And topping the list of risk factors is a sedentary lifestyle. That is why cardiologists are convinced that the *best "cure" for heart disease is the preventive medicine known as exercise*. It is why they advise taking your circulatory system for a brisk walk or a jog or a swim or a session of leaf-raking on a regular basis.

Beating Back Pain

Here's another benefit of exercise—it helps prevent back pain.

Research confirms that people who exercise regularly have far fewer back problems than those who lead a sedentary lifestyle. When the muscles surrounding the joint between your lumbar vertebrae and your sacrum get out of condition—as they will without exercise—they can no longer protect your lower back, which becomes the weak link in your body's support system. Lifting or bending becomes painful, and you can easily "pull out" your back—a painful and debilitating condition. Recent studies have shown that when you do "pull out" your back, light exercise is the cure—as well as the prevention.

Exercising Intelligently

Studies on animals show that *aerobic exercise* doesn't just improve cardiovascular health, but also *aids the brain, promoting the generation of new brain cells*, called neurons, and of the connections between them, synapses. In short, the more we walk, run, leap, play tennis, swim—whatever—the more efficient and adaptive our brains become, and the less susceptible to age-related downslides.

And you don't need to become a gym rat to reap all the benefits of exercise. What seems to stop a lot of people from exercising is the notion that they have to spend a lot of time on it. On a hectic schedule, many people figure they don't have hours to spare for gym workouts. No matter how you slice it, getting to a gym or health club cuts almost two hours out of your day—what with getting there, changing, the postworkout shower, and so on. But recent studies now tell us that the single, long exercise workout may not be as effective in terms of heart health as three daily ten-minute sessions of moderate intensity.

By "moderate intensity," the study authors mean a brisk walk or an easy jog—enough to burn a total of about 250 calories. One study, performed at Southwest Missouri State University, found that the rise in blood fats after meals was less pronounced after intermittent exercise than after continuous exercise—and certainly than after no exercise at all. Participants in the study were actually people who did not exercise regularly.

Bottom line? You don't need a gym membership, workout suit, gym bag, or other accessories to get fit. If you don't have the time for sustained exercise, take ten to walk briskly up the office stairs, or park at the far end of the mall parking lot and jog to the store.

Exercise for Diabetics

Physicians estimate that by changing eating habits and undertaking a regular program of exercise, three-fourths of today's diabetes patients could safely and beneficially stop using medication. Aerobic exercise can decrease insulin requirements by 30 percent to 50 percent for Type I diabetes and by up to 100 percent for Type II diabetes.

A Doctor's Favorite Recommendation

Given all these benefits, is it any wonder that doctors recommend exercise? In fact, it's the perfect health prescription—all pluses, with no ill side effects. And it's a universal healer. No matter your fitness condition or your physical limitations, there is some form of activity you can do.

So my prescription—and I doubt there's a doctor anywhere who wouldn't sign on to this same Rx—is this: Where physical activity is concerned, do more of it, and do it more often. Your overall health will be enhanced, and just about any health ailment you may have will improve as a result.

Since this is the case, and since everyone knows that physical activity is something that will improve their lives in every way, what is the problem? Why doesn't everyone exercise all the time? Why do patients tell me about the many exercise programs they have begun and then abandoned? About the treadmill in the bedroom that serves as a clothes rack? About the tennis racket/jogging shoes/swim fins—you name it—they purchased at great expense and with great resolve that now languish in the back of a closet?

Maybe we hear too much about exercise and its benefits. Maybe the whole subject has been made much more complicated than it needs to be. Let me simplify, and that will give you a hint of what the next eleven days are going to be about.

I'll start with this statement, put as simply as possible: ***To move is to live***, and the more you move, the healthier and longer your life will be.

Here's another simple statement: ***The more you do, the more you can do***—and the longer you can do it for.

Now let me put both statements together and make it simpler still: Physical activity is a sign of life. The more physical activity you do, the more life your life will have—and the longer it will last.

Get ready to liberate your body, enhance your physical and emotional and spiritual strength, feel empowered, strengthen your immune system, and take your life to a whole new level of energy, health, ability, and possibility.

That is what exercise will do for you. And that is why I ask you to do it well. Concentrate. Focus. Work with your body in space to reenergize yourself. And challenge your limits. Believe me when I say that you can. After all, you put the limits there; with the physical activity you are about to undertake, you can pull them down.

Looking Forward to the Next Eleven Days

No wonder, then, that exercise is one of the essential elements of my eleven-day life-expansion plan. As usual, the first four days will help you develop your awareness while the final seven days will put your plan into action.

Awareness and action go hand in hand. That is, it may be hard to imagine yourself doing a whole lot of things until you actually get up and get moving. For that reason, I'm urging you to start taking action from the first day of this program. It's the simplest type of action you can imagine—that is, just walking. But in the time you spend walking, during the first four days, you will also start building your awareness of what you can do—and how.

On the third day, I want you to continue walking, but also expand your knowledge of exercises. In one section at the end of this chapter, I have asked experts to describe their favorite exercise programs, including **yoga**, **Pilates**, **tai chi**, **Body Rolling**, **Core Fusion**, the **Picture Perfect Prescription for exercise**, and a number of others. I'd like you to learn something about each of those different kinds of exercise programs because one or more of them might be just right for you.

We picked several different areas of exercise routines because each one of them offers different benefits. Some are more difficult, while others are easier. But there are other distinctions as well. *Some have a spiritual component*, giving you a feeling of calm, while *others will push you to maximum activity and physical exertion.*

On the fourth day of awareness building, I'll ask you to choose one—and sign up for it. But before you get to that point, you'll want to read the sections at the end of this chapter and follow some of the demonstrations included on the DVD. That way, you'll know what's involved in each type of exercise program, how much commitment it takes, and what the benefits are. Believe me, with all the opportunities that are available, exercise never needs to be dull.

Exercise Hang-ups

So what is it that keeps people from doing some form of exercise on a regular basis? Why does something that begins with enthusiasm and vows of eternal commitment dribble down to a hit-or-miss proposition? I've known patients who expend significant time and energy rationalizing why they can't exercise today. If only they'd apply half that effort to the exercise itself they'd be far better off!

Do you feel that you have to make a vow of commitment to a particular program? I know that does hang some people up. They think they have to purchase expensive gear, mark a start date on the calendar, and throw themselves into a program with new enthusiasm. In other words, they regard an exercise program as a break from the norm.

When people approach an exercise program with this attitude, I am reminded of the mind-set that so many bring to diets. They're set up like special-training programs, isolated from daily life. But if you approach a program that way, it's bound to feel like something temporary.

As with diets, ***one reason exercise programs often fail is that they too often deviate from the norm rather than becoming the norm***. Unless physical activity becomes a habitual part of your daily life—until it is so woven into the fabric of your routine that it cannot be separated—then no amount of flashy gear or vows of commitment will get you up, out, and moving every day.

Another problem: Some people undertake an exercise program for the same reason they try out a trendy new restaurant. Rather than discovering and savoring their personal preferences, they gravitate toward the same fitness routines or exercises that other people favor. Years ago, jogging was all the rage—till it yielded to power walking. Then came "spinning" on stationary bicycles, closely followed by circuit training, yoga, and Pilates. I don't know what the exercise flavor of the month will be by the time this book is published, but I do know that the right program for you is the one that you choose yourself. In exercise, as in everything else, fashions change pretty rapidly. Too often, people take up an exercise that simply doesn't fit their physical needs, physical condition, fitness level, or interest. Pretty soon, doing the exercise program, fashionable though it may be, becomes a chore. It becomes a chore you increasingly put off doing. And finally, it becomes a memory.

It's natural to be intrigued by the latest fashion. But when you know what fits you most comfortably, you'll always come back to it in the end. Besides, starting an exercise program because it's in style seems the wrong way to go about it. Shouldn't your exercise program start with you—your needs, your fitness level, and what you hope to achieve by exercising?

Psychological Benefits of Physical Activity

- Decreased stress, tension, and anxiety
- Improved self-confidence and body image
- Enhanced mood
- Prevention/alleviation of depression
- Increased mental alertness

So where exercise hang-ups are concerned, the bottom line is this: *The physical activity you undertake has to be something that fits your life and your lifestyle. It should be something you enjoy.* Only then will you successfully integrate it into your days, weeks, and months—for the rest of your life.

That is why a very important part of this eleven-day program will be about figuring out what kinds of exercise can work for you—what kinds of exercise meet your needs and offer sufficient satisfaction or enjoyment. It will also be about understanding that as your needs change and your interests shift, you can and must find new kinds of exercise to do so that you keep moving and remain active for life.

The best thing you can do over these next eleven days is make a transition from a life of hit-or-miss exercise, or none at all, to a life of regular physical activity. Use the time to honestly assess the kind of physical activity you want to do, need to do, and will feel comfortable doing. Then go out and do it—for life.

MOVE

THE ELEVEN-DAY PROGRAM

DAYS 1–4: THE AWARENESS DAYS

In these first four days, I'm going to ask you to do a lot of thinking, a fair amount of list-making, and as much self-motivating as you need. But as I mentioned previously, I am going to ask you to do all this while you're walking. So on each of these first four days, there will be some exercise time (walking) followed by some writing time.

Why does every doctor recommend walking? Simply because there is no better exercise than putting one foot in front of the other. The latest research on *walking* as exercise—at a brisk pace, with arms pumping—shows that it *can lower the risk of heart disease by as much as 30 percent.* Walking *strengthens bones, improves the functioning of all the organs, enhances the immune system, clears cobwebs from the brain, and lifts your mood.*

Furthermore, it's low-tech. The only equipment you need is a comfortable pair of shoes and clothing appropriate for the weather. (In fact, even weather doesn't have to be a factor, since there are so many indoor malls where people can walk.) Unless you are severely restricted by a medical condition, anyone and everyone can walk. It costs nothing.

During the next four days, choose a walking terrain wherever you like—on city streets, along country roads, in a mall, or even on a treadmill. For maximum benefit, you want to include an uphill climb somewhere along your route. (If you're doing most of your walking indoors, make sure that you walk up at least three flights of steps at some point.) Start at a comfortable pace, ease into it for the first minute or minute and a half, and by minute two, you should be at a brisk pace that you maintain steadily.

As you'll see on Days 1 through 4, I recommend that you measure your walks in time rather than by distance. Start with fifteen minutes on Day 1, then put in some additional walking time every day. While the walking should be brisk—more than a stroll—there's no reason to break into a running pace.

What constitutes brisk walking? The rule of thumb is to assume a pace such that you'll cover a mile in about twenty minutes. As walking becomes a daily habit, you might improve to a fifteen-minute mile. Just walk at a good clip, fast enough that you feel the effort. If you're going so fast that you can't talk to a companion without huffing and puffing between sentences, then you need to slow down.

Day 1: Determine what shape you are in.
Today:
- Walk twenty minutes.
- Evaluate your level of fitness and physical condition.

I will bet my New York practice that when you saw those words "what shape you are in," "level of fitness," and "physical condition," your mind immediately began to catalog your aches and pains. You were ready to relate that you feel stiff when you get out of bed in the morning, or that your joints hurt, or that you're overweight, or that this walk is making you short of breath. You were all set to complain that as you walk uphill, your thigh muscles seem to scream their resistance, and that as you walk downhill, your knees creak.

You know what? Everybody's knees creak. Everybody gets short of breath. Everybody feels a little stiff after being in one place for a while. So forget your inadequacies; they're old news, and they're universal.

What I want you to concentrate on instead is what's *right* about your body. Tell me about your good points. Keep in mind that I don't want to hear what other people have told you about the shape you're in, and I certainly don't want to hear what you've internalized from what society thinks constitutes the "right" shape. Instead, as you walk today, as you stride forward with your arms swinging, I want you to be reminded of how strong you are. It is that strength we are going to build on during this eleven-day program, and it is important for you to know your starting point.

There are two things I want you to concentrate on:

- First, **add up your body's pluses**—your physical strengths and best features.
- Then, **think about what you love to do physically**—the work or play or effort or energy expenditure that makes you feel good, powerful, and most alive.

Start with the body's pluses. Focus on the positive. For instance, here are some of the attributes that you might want to list:

- I am stronger than anyone would suspect.
- I have a very nice butt.
- I have shapely arms.
- I have as much energy and stamina as a kid.
- I look great in stiletto heels.

In the same spirit, name the physical things you've done that you've found to be thrilling. List things that got your heart racing—emotionally as well as physiologically. Here are some ideas to get you started:

- I like to hike in the mountains.
- That time I tried snowboarding, I really enjoyed it.
- I remember the day I painted the spare bedroom all by myself—exhausting but rewarding!
- I had a great time helping the neighbor dig a new garden.

Remember all the things you've done recently or in the past

that made you feel good in your body, even though you were tired or even achy afterward.

When you get home from the walk, get out a pad of paper. On one sheet, *write the heading* "My body's strengths and best features." *On a second sheet*, write "The activities that make me feel physically good." Try to fill up both sheets—and use more—recalling what you thought about during your walk, then adding even more.

Take a look at what you've written. It's a lot to be excited about. And that's where we start.

Results of Day 1: *You've found your starting point—and you're ready to go forward from there.*

Day 2: *What do you want exercise to do for you?*
Today:
- Walk twenty minutes.
- Think about what you want to do with a stronger, more powerful, more capable body.

I want you to concentrate on the things you're going to achieve with a regimen of physical activity. As you're walking, here are some questions to ask yourself.
- Do I want more energy?
- Would I like to lose weight and gain endurance?
- Would I like the chance to shop in a store I've never dared go into because the styles and sizes were "all wrong" for me?
- Do I want to improve my performance in a sport?
- Would I like to be able to bend, lift, and carry without feeling pain?
- Am I tired of feeling tired all the time?

- Would I like to look better?
- Is it my goal to stave off disease?
- Do I have a more specific goal—like wanting to run a marathon, climb Mount Kilimanjaro, or beat my fifteen-year-old daughter in tennis?
- Would I like to leap out of bed every morning feeling like I'm eager to start the day?
- Do I want to avoid the heart attack my mother had?
- Do I want to play a better game of golf by next summer?

Whatever your aim or aims—you may certainly have more than one—it's important to articulate what you hope to gain for yourself by making physical activity a part of your life. So when you get home from your walk, make a third list in addition to the two that you created yesterday. *At the head of this sheet of paper, write* "What I want to achieve with physical activity." *Then list all the places you want your body to take you and all the powers you want it to possess.*

Results of Day 2: *You've defined your goals by naming what you want to achieve when you make physical activity a part of your life.*

Medical Benefits of Aerobic Exercise

When you're making your list of goals, consider some of the proven health benefits of regular exercise. Here are just some of them:

- Increased maximal oxygen consumption
- Improved heart and lung function
  - o More blood pumped every minute
  - o More blood pumped with each heartbeat
  - o Increased ability to carry oxygen
  - o Reduced workload on the heart
- Increased blood supply to muscles and ability to use oxygen
- Lower heart rate and blood pressure at any level of exercise
- Increased threshold for lactic acid accumulation
- Lower resting systolic and diastolic blood pressure in people with high blood pressure
- Increased HDL cholesterol (the good cholesterol)
- Decreased blood triglycerides
- Reduced body fat and improved weight control
- Improved glucose tolerance and reduced insulin resistance

Day 3: *What kind of exercise do you prefer?*
Today:
- Walk for a half hour.
- Consider the kinds of physical activity available to you—and select the ones that are most appealing.

As you walk a full half hour today, I want you to choose which avenue of physical activity you want to follow. The idea is to undertake a program of physical activity that has significant benefits, but without adding a lot of psychological burdens to your life.

If you find a particular form of exercise boring or embarrassing, for example, why try to pursue it? The chances are good you won't stick with it. Instead, I'd like you to consider your inclinations, quirks, likes, and dislikes at the outset. Be selective. First, consider the variety of activities that are available. After that, you can make a match that works.

Basically, *all forms of exercise fall into one of three categories—sport and recreation, lifestyle exercise,* and *structured programs.*

Sports and recreational exercise are the most common forms of activity, but often, people approach sports a lot more competitively. If you really pursue a sport—trying to cycle the way Lance Armstrong does, for example—it can become intense. But there's also the recreational form of cycling, the way a couple or family might do it on the weekend, following a trail or quiet country lane. Similarly, tennis, basketball, or baseball can be highly competitive sports, but you can also enjoy them as regular recreation. On the recreation side, don't forget activities like ballroom dancing or jumping rope. These are just a few of the aerobic exercises that particularly benefit heart and lungs.

Are You Ready?

Consider the following list, and put a checkmark beside any activity that you've tried in the past. Then put a double-check next to the ones that you've never tried—but would like to. Are there other activities that you've tried in the past or would like to pursue? Which ones would you add to this list?

Ballroom dancing ____   Square dancing ____
Ballet ____   Volleyball ____
Weight training ____   Softball ____
Tennis ____   Tap dancing ____
Horseback riding ____   Ice skating ____
Synchronized swimming ____   Running ____
Spelunking ____   Golf ____
Pilates ____   Body Rolling ____
Racquetball ____   Cycling ____
Fencing ____   Handball ____
Yoga ____   Kickboxing ____
Tai chi ____   Jumping rope ____
Line dancing ____   Hiking ____
Archery ____   Basketball ____
Soccer ____   Core Fusion ____
Flamenco ____   Belly dancing ____
In-line skating ____   Squash ____
Rope climbing ____   Baseball ____

Your additions

_____

_____

_____

_____

Lifestyle exercises are the many physical activities you can do at home or in the course of the day to gain benefits of both aerobic exercise and weight training. Vacuuming the house, weeding the garden, walking the dog, washing the car, cleaning the basement, raking leaves—all these are significant calorie-burning aerobics that strengthen musculature, bone, and tissue. So it's a good idea to do more housework if you can, not less.

You can add to the range and benefits of lifestyle exercise by making certain choices. To name a few:

- If you live or work in a building serviced by an elevator, take the stairs whenever possible.
- When driving to a mall or supermarket, don't cruise around looking for the nearest parking space—instead, park as far away as possible and walk to your destination.
- If you have a lawn to mow, use a push mower—better yet, a reel mower without an engine—rather than a sit-down mower.

In other words, whenever you can, avoid the technologically advanced convenience in favor of expending a little more effort. If you consistently follow a pattern of seeking more exercise, not less, you will soon see and feel the difference without any extra effort at all.

The structured programs that I've described in the second part of this chapter give you a wide variety to choose from. Each of these programs is introduced by a single expert, and *you'll find further instructions and demonstrations on the DVD* that accompanies this book. Here are six programs you can choose from:

1. The ancient practice of *yoga* is known for keeping the body supple and limber. But *yoga* also gives "a boost to the system," says yoga teacher Michael Lechonczak. It conditions the spirit as well as the body and engenders a sense of connectedness

that can be both "soothing and healing."

2. A ***combination of Pilates and dance***, created by Ron Fletcher, starts in the body's center, nurtures the total body, and is aimed at letting "everyone realize all the potential of their own body, mind, breath, and spirit."

3. ***Body Rolling***, invented by Yamuna Zake, is all about bringing the body back into alignment so that everything works better. "You don't have to accept limitations on your mobility and on feeling good," Yamuna tells us in an interview. With her Body Rolling system, you "can liberate and lift your body and give it room and space to function."

4. Lawrence Tan's twenty-first-century version of the ancient Chinese practice of ***tai chi*** brings this "moving meditation" into the lives of even the most pressed-for-time contemporary individuals. Using Tan's tai chi methods, you can discover how to move the body, concentrate the mind, and breathe to "achieve a centered, calm state of mind and being."

5. ***Core Fusion***, which is perhaps the latest entry in the structured-exercise-program stakes, fuses yoga, Pilates, orthopedic, and core conditioning exercises. Core Fusion strives to "restore and maintain the balance between strength and flexibility," according to its creator, Fred DeVito. When you've been doing Core Fusion exercises, you're left with what DeVito calls a "calm energy."

6. You can create your own ***personal training program*** by combining these and many other exercises. This Picture Perfect Prescription Program is demonstrated by personal trainer Heather Raymond. Her guidelines and demonstrations will help you choose an exercise program that's

designed to take you along the right path of physical activity. "When you are exercising," says Raymond, "you are taking active control of your health, and that improves your overall quality of life."

As you review these activities and make a list of things you'd like to do, be sensible. Discard those options you know you are unlikely ever to undertake. Then make room for those activities you have perhaps secretly always wanted to try. Push the envelope.

Results of Day 3: *You have looked at the options and chosen exercises that seem just right for your body and your temperament.*

Day 4: Make a calendar of your exercise commitment.

Today:

- Walk forty-five minutes.
- Put your plan into action—with a call and a calendar.

During your walk today, I want you to resolve an initial program of regular physical activity. And by the end of the day, you need to "sign on" to that program.

When I say "sign on," I mean it literally. Just saying to yourself that you're really going to start exercising this time is not sufficient. There must be some concrete sign of your commitment.

Let me give you an example. As you're walking, consider how much you've enjoyed your daily walks. Perhaps what you'd like to do for your exercise program is continue the walks you've been doing. If so, make a calendar on which you jot down the number of minutes you're going to walk each day. Put that calendar on the refrigerator or bathroom mirror—someplace where you'll see it daily.

Some other possible action steps:

- Suppose you've decided on ballroom dancing. The next step is to get a partner and plan your evenings of dancing, or sign up for classes.
- If your choice is tennis, sign up for lessons or reserve a court and schedule games with an opponent.
- If you've decided to opt for lifestyle exercises, make a to-do list of the ones you'll finish this week—such as cleaning the attic, mowing the lawn, or organizing the garage.
- If your choice is a team sport, make a call and get on a team.
- If you have chosen a structured program, sign up.

You've spent four days assessing your physical fitness and thinking how you can best improve it. Today, make a tangible commitment to that improvement.

Results of Day 4: *You have a calendar of exercise that you'll look forward to doing in the days ahead.*

Days 5–11: The Action Days

In the next week, I want you to follow a number of action steps: they make up the ***Picture Perfect Prescription seven-day sampler***. Now that you have made some choices about the kind of physical activity you want to commit to for the long term, you'll want to try these brief, simple exercises that use every bit of your body. The exercises you'll learn over the next seven days will help build upper-body strength, lower-body strength, core strength, and total body strength. Whatever kind of exercise program you've chosen for the long term—sports and recreation, lifestyle, or structured—this seven-day sampler will give you additional guidance to improve flexibility and build strength. On days when you can't follow your regular program of exercise, use this prescription as a backup, so you'll stay in the habit of exercise every day.

You'll learn and do one exercise per day. When you have sampled all seven, you can put them together for a workout of your own. Use each as needed.

Ready? Let's begin.

Strength Training Tips

If you decide to implement a strength-training program after the Picture-Perfect Prescription Seven-Day Sampler, keep in mind that the goal is to build muscle in order to accelerate your metabolism, enhance your resilience and response to potential injury, and tone your appearance. Remember that muscles grow when you work them really hard—and then rest them adequately. For that reason, take a rest day between strength workouts. Do an upper body workout one day, then have a rest day, then do your lower body, then have another rest day, then the core exercises followed by a rest day. The rest days will enable you to work "to failure" when you do work out so that you maximize your exercise program.

As you grow fitter and your workouts become more intense, you should leave even more time between strength sessions on a particular muscle group—two days instead of one, for example. On these "off" days, go for a brisk walk, do some stretching, or pursue a sport activity.

And don't worry that heavy weights will make you "bulk up." On the contrary. The fact is that muscle tissue takes up one third the space of fat tissue, and as you add muscle tissue, you will eventually lose stored body fat and end up tighter and more toned—not bulky. But don't add weight to your workout at the expense of form. Best is to go slowly and keep your motions deliberate and controlled. Be there! Good luck.

Strength-Training Strengths

Strong muscle means strong bones, so when we begin to lose about a quarter pound of muscle every year starting in our late thirties or early forties, it's serious. That's why it's so important to work our muscles to keep them strong, and the most effective way to do that is with weight training.

There are other reasons to do weight training besides just trying to keep up with our muscle loss. For one thing, if we don't activate our muscles, the muscle cells begin to resist the insulin that the pancreas secretes, giving us a higher risk of heart disease and diabetes.

In addition, of course, muscle burns more calories than fat does. More muscle means a higher metabolic rate, which makes it easier to stay slim. Here are some of the direct health benefits of strength training:

- Increased muscular strength
- Increased strength of tendons and ligaments
- Improved flexibility—i.e., range of motion of joints
- Reduced body fat and increased muscle mass
- Potentially decreased resting systolic and diastolic blood pressure
- Positive changes in blood cholesterol
- Improved glucose tolerance and insulin sensitivity
- Improved strength, balance, and functional ability in older adults

(Continued from page 96)

To be sure, aerobic training—or any exercise program, for that matter—can help you lose weight, but strength training provides the firmness that so improves people's appearance—and their self-esteem.

Perhaps above all, as we age, strong muscles can mean mobility and independence—as well as feeling and looking good.

The bottom line? Strength training offers phenomenal benefits for health, youthfulness, and staving off the debilitating effects of aging.

Day 5: *Do push-ups to help develop upper-body strength.*

I am not going to ask you to drop down and give me twenty. Instead, you'll be asked to do push-ups correctly, in good form.

There are two ways to do these push-ups. If you have enough upper-body strength, you can do a classic push-up, raising your whole body onto your hands and toes. But there's also a modified form—pushing up from your knees. Whichever kind you do, it's important to keep form while you're doing the push-ups. That is, try to keep your head, shoulders, torso, and legs aligned just as shown in the illustrations. When you have to struggle to raise yourself and can no longer keep form, that's a sign that it's time to stop or take a break.

Here's how to do the classic push-up:

Position your body facedown on the floor. Bring your hands out perpendicular from your sides so that your upper arms are at a right angle to the floor. Tuck your toes under.

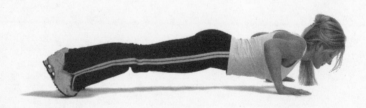

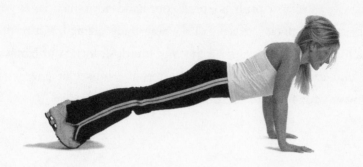

Now tense up your legs—keeping them as straight as possible—as you push into the floor with your hands and lift your upper body. Do not lock your elbows, and do not stick your backside up in the air. Keep your body in one long line from your nose to your toes.

Hold, then lower as slowly as possible. If you can stop halfway to the floor, push up again from the halfway point. If not, slowly lower yourself to the floor, then push up again. Pay attention to your form.

Repeat the push-ups until you can no longer keep form.

The second way to do push-ups is in the modified form, lifting yourself from the knees rather than toes. Begin in the bent-knee position shown.

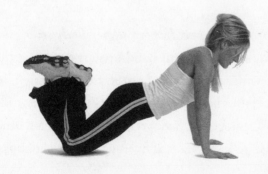

As with the classic push-up, press your hands into the floor as you straighten your elbows. Keep your whole body aligned, with your stomach tight. Raise yourself all the way, but don't lock your elbows.

If you can, stop halfway down—feel the muscular energy; if not, lower your body to the floor between push-ups.

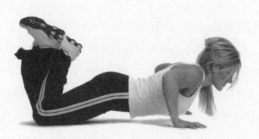

Whichever style you choose, do push-ups to the point of failure, as fitness professionals call it—which simply means do it until you can no longer push up *with proper form.*

Results of Day 5: *You have mastered an exercise to develop upper-body strength.*

Day 6: Do dips to further develop upper body strength.

Start by sitting on your hands, palms down, on the edge of a stable chair, with your feet well out in front of you.

With your elbows behind you, roll your shoulders back and squeeze the shoulder blades together. Slide your butt off the chair, bending your knees, and begin to lower yourself by using your upper arms.

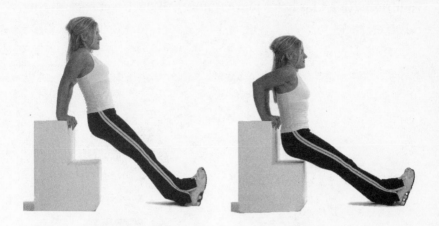

When you have lowered yourself to the position shown (or as close as possible), hold for a moment. Then slowly raise yourself back up, using the strength of your upper arms.

To make this exercise more challenging, straighten your legs out in front of you, balancing on your heels.

Do these dips to the point of failure or exhaustion—that is, till you can no longer keep form.

Results of Day 6: *You have now mastered a second exercise to improve upper-body strength.*

Day 7: Practice squats to develop lower-body strength.

For this exercise, you will need dumbbells or some other kind of weight that you can easily hold in both hands. Starting weights should not be heavy—five or ten pounds is usually enough. If you don't have dumbbells, you can use books (just make sure they're both the same weight) or plastic containers that are partially filled with water.

Hold the weights as shown. Position yourself with your toes

pointing forward and feet placed shoulder width apart. Pull in your stomach. (This helps prevent injury to the lower back during this exercise.)

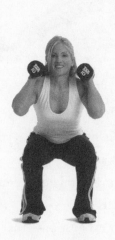
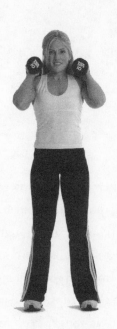

Shift your butt backward and bend at the knees until your thighs are parallel to the floor. Hold.

Now straighten your knees and return to a standing position.

Repeat as many times as you can without losing form.

Results of Day 7: *You have mastered a key exercise for improving lower-body strength.*

Day 8: Learn how to do side lunges for lower-body strength.

Stand facing forward, holding a weight as shown.

Lift your left leg and lunge to the left. At the end of the move, your left foot should be pointing forward. The right foot remains pointing forward.

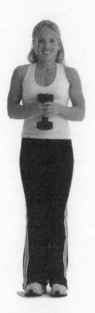
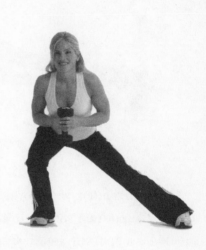

Now flex the right knee and lower your body until your right thigh is parallel to the floor. Hold.

Press your right foot into the floor and push off. At the end of this move, you should be standing upright with both feet together again.

Now repeat the exercise, lunging to the right.

Alternate left and right lunges.

Try to do twenty per side.

Results of Day 8: *You have mastered side lunges for lower-body strength.*

Day 9: Do the plank for core-body strength.

Position yourself on a rug or exercise mat as shown.

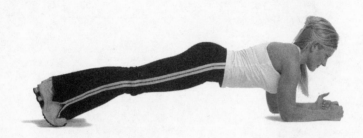

Now straighten your torso and extend your legs until you assume the position shown. In this posture, your elbows and toes should be supporting your body.

Hold the pose, keeping your body in one long, straight line from nose to toes—like a plank. Hold as long as you can. You should be able to feel muscle tension all along your body.

Results of Day 9: *You have learned a daily exercise for core-body strength.*

Day 10: Practice opposite arm and leg extensions.

Get down on all fours on a soft rug or mat. Position yourself so your neck is aligned with your back and you're looking down at the floor.

Lift and extend your left arm and right leg simultaneously until both are parallel to the floor. Try to hold for a count of three.

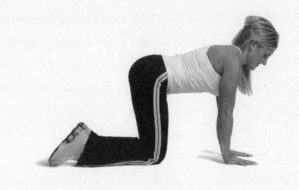

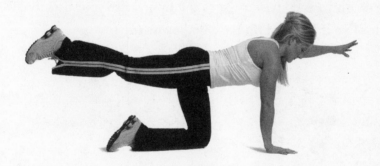

Return your arm and leg to the starting position.

Now lift and extend your right arm and left leg simultaneously. Again, hold for at least three seconds.

Try to do twenty of these extensions, alternating left and right.

Results of Day 10: *You have mastered a second exercise for core body strength.*

Day 11: Learn the power punch.

Today, you'll be doing an exercise that requires strength, balance, and energy. To begin, take a fighting stance, as shown. Your feet should be shoulder-width apart, with one foot slightly forward of the other.

The forward foot is the one on the nondominant side of your body—that is, left foot if you are right-handed and the right foot if you are left-handed. Your dominant-side foot should be about 10 inches back. Rise up on the ball of that foot.

Be sure to hold a position such that your left foot is under the left shoulder and right foot is under the right shoulder. Your knees should be bent, with weight distributed evenly between both feet.

With your body squared to the front, raise your fists to either side of your face and tip the chin downward.

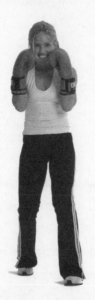 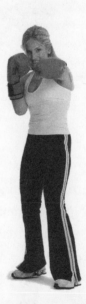

The first move of the power punch is the jab. From the fighting stance, lead with your nondominant hand—that is, the hand on the same side as the forward leg. Thrust your fist out straight, twisting the fist as you thrust so that the palm faces downward at "impact." As you thrust, turn your body slightly away from the punch for leverage, keeping your feet pointing forward.

Exhale as you thrust. Power the jab from the legs and midsection. Don't use just your arms. And never lock or hyperextend the joints. Pull the fist back.

Now try the cross. From the fighting stance, lead with your dominant hand—the one on the same side as the back leg. Thrust straight out, as in the jab, and rotate the fist so that it ends up parallel to the floor, palm down, as in the jab. But this time, as you throw the punch, twist the hips away from the punch. At the same time, twist the back foot on the floor as if you were putting out a cigarette; this provides additional power to the punch.

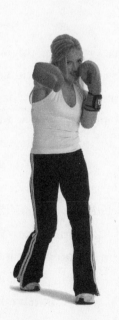

Exhale as you throw a cross. Again, the punch is being thrown by the body rather than by the arm. Bring it back.

Put the two punches together. Jab with your nondominant hand, then follow it quickly with a hard cross, twisting the hips and following through with the shoulder and the rest of the body. Punch from the midsection and legs, where your greatest power resides.

Results of Day 11: *With this exercise, an energy explosion puts your entire body in motion.*

GET UP, GET OUT, GET MOVING:
THE STRUCTURED PROGRAMS

If you become familiar with structured programs and exercise regimens, you will discover that you have an almost limitless number of options to choose from. To introduce you to these, *I have chosen renowned practitioners of six of the most exciting and beneficial programs I have seen. In addition to what you read in this book, you will find supplementary information from these leading experts—along with some demonstrations—on the DVD that's provided.*

YOGA
Michael Lechonczak

The practice of yoga is so ancient that its actual origins are shrouded in mystery. What is certain, however, is that for thousands of years, yoga has been transforming lives and bringing the balm of relaxation, the benefits of physical strength and suppleness, and, in many cases, a sense of spiritual harmony to millions all over the world. Just ask Michael Lechonczak.

Lechonczak was, by his own admission, a "stressed-out office manager and administrator" who finally decided to try meditation as a way to deal with his "jangled and agitated" state. When someone told him yoga could be helpful in learning meditation, Lechonczak went along to a yoga class—and changed his life forever. "I found myself going through various levels of relaxation," he recalls of that first class. "I experienced an immediate soothing and healing and felt an enormous sense of relief. It was a very powerful experience for me."

It all "felt so good and delicious" that Lechonczak began doing yoga on a regular basis, sampling the wide variety of practice styles. As his consciousness about yoga increased, his job satisfaction decreased, and when he was caught in a corporate downsizing, he was able to see the end of office life as a gift—a chance to pursue what he really wanted to do: yoga. In time and after significant study, Lechonczak became a yoga teacher in his own right. Today, he teaches in a well-known New York health club, serves a select private clientele, and, with his wife, also a yoga teacher, offers yoga retreats all over the world.

The Path of Yoga

"There are as many styles of yoga as there are models of cars," Lechonczak says, "but they all derive from hatha yoga, which is the physical practice of postures, *asana*s, and breath work, *pranayama*." The postures and breath work together become a path along which it may be possible to integrate mind, body, and spirit—a wholeness that is both physical and spiritual.

As exercise, yoga has the effect of keeping the body supple and limber for a lifetime. "In effect," says Lechonczak, "doing yoga is physical multitasking. You're working all sorts of muscle groups in different ways. You might be strengthening one set of muscles while lengthening another set of muscles while also amplifying your breath work."

The aim is "to work the body intelligently." That means to come into the particular posture with the right form, with alignment— that is, with awareness that the bones are lined up, that the joints are in the right place, that the muscles are correctly supporting the joints and skeletal structure. When you're in alignment in this way, blood flows more easily, which means more oxygen throughout the body, which in turn means more nutrients and more energy.

"With the body in alignment," Lechonczak continues, "you increase the space in the joints. The joints are no longer being crushed or twisted. In a very real sense, you have created space in the body. Even fractions of space can be crucial; they can mean the difference between pain and having a normal life. It is all a matter of alignment."

Take the case of the spine. Says Lechonczak: "We say that you're as young as your spine. If your spine is calcified and immobile, you're old. If your spine is supple, flexible, open, you're young regardless of your age. That's one of the key ideas of yoga. And yoga always lengthens the spine, constantly creating more space between vertebrae.

"Again, this facilitates vascularity—widened blood vessels for better blood flow—so that everything in the body functions more efficiently. The nerves that emanate from the spinal column are no longer impinged; that's what happens when you compress those nerves: you pinch them, and it's very painful. Yoga lengthens the spine, opens up that compression."

Conditioning Both Body and Spirit

All of the numerous postures of yoga produce similar benefits. "Do a twist correctly," says Lechonczak, "with proper form and alignment, and you are aware that you are squeezing deoxygenated blood and toxins out of your internal organs. Then, as you release the twist, fresh blood rushes in. The posture training makes the body better able to process the blood and recondition it. It's an enormous boost to the total system."

As to the different styles of yoga—hot yoga, power yoga, and the like—Lechonczak simply cautions that people must follow a style that is appropriate for their conditioning and their lifestyle. He advises people to define the results that they seek and, above all, choose yoga exercises—or a type of yoga—that won't cause injury. "Some styles are right for conditioned young athletes, but not for deconditioned fifty-year-olds. All the styles have their merits. The point is to find the practice that's right for you in terms of conditioning and the results you are looking for."

Whatever type of yoga you choose to do, Lechonczak advocates a meditative approach. In his instructions, he focuses on physical positioning, but it's always combined with attention to details that include attentiveness, awareness, and breathing as well as posture. For instance, consider his instructions for a single posture, the warrior pose: "Take a step, put your knee precisely here, let your attention move over your back leg, use your thigh muscles to lift the flesh above the kneecap, breathe fully and consciously." The point is clearly and dramatically drawn: in achieving such a posture, "we bring people into their bodies and breath so as to allow them to connect, to be absolutely present. The slightest possibility of anxiety just drops away. The mind stops wandering: you're *in* your body, *in* your breath, and you're getting a nonimpact workout that will keep you supple for life."

For many, of course, yoga goes beyond the meditative to the spiritual. "When you integrate body, mind, and breath," says Lechonczak, "this equates to a spiritual experience." Stress, anxiety, anger, resentment melt away—replaced by a feeling of peace, a sense of wholeness, and a sensation of connectedness.

See the demonstration on the DVD.

BODY ROLLING
Yamuna Zake

"Being fit is about aligning the body. There is a natural order in the body, and when it is properly aligned, with everything in its optimal place, then you are strong, your organs function better, your muscles hold you up. Your body is working at its full potential—and you look it."

So says Yamuna Zake, creator of Yamuna Body Logic and Yamuna Body Rolling, a unique kind of self-therapy. As demonstrated on the DVD, her exercises are done with a plastic ball. As you roll the ball over different parts of your body, you elongate the muscles, stimulate the bone and organs, free the connective tissue, and strengthen and tone the total body.

"We all misalign our bodies," Yamuna asserts. "From the time we are little and are told to sit up straight or be careful, we are always gripping and tightening. Then we grow up and sit at a desk all day, where our hip joints get tight and our abdominal muscles get soft, and circulation to our organs gets cut off so our organs slow down. Our body starts letting us down: our feet hurt, we have neck pain, we wake up in the morning and our muscles are stiff. We feel lousy. We also look lousy. When you have droopy posture, that's how people perceive you."

In some cases, says Yamuna, exercising can actually make you even more tense, tight, and prone to injury. "If you do the treadmill every day but do it with bad posture," she explains, "you could be setting yourself up for an injury which can then sabotage your attempts at fitness."

Unless we correct the misalignment, it grows more pronounced as we get older—to the point that it can restrict us from doing what we want to do. Yamuna also makes the point that you can't wait until retirement to begin working on body alignment and flexibility. Her exercises are designed so you can begin now—no matter what your daily occupation or where you work.

Yamuna's Body Logic and Body Rolling therapy are all about getting your body aligned and keeping it working and in shape. The program supports any kind of exercise workout, sport, or activity, for as long as you live. And it helps to extend life because your body simply functions better.

Getting Unstuck and Aligned

The objective is to return our bodies to their optimal functioning, with every organ in its optimal place. How does it work? How does rolling a ball along our bodies give us back our natural alignment?

"Basically, it is about letting go," says Yamuna. "It's about lifting, releasing, and stimulating every part of the body to give back the space each needs."

Just as a piece of cloth can become folded in a way that changes the shape of the garment, so with the body. And just as you can iron out the crease in a blouse, so can you iron out the creases in the body. When you do—essentially by smoothing out the creases—you get back the space that had been wrinkled.

The plastic balls that Yamuna designed are unique. (For information on how to order them, see the "Resources" section.) As you roll the ball along one part of your body, its pressure and motion helps to elongate the muscles. Essentially, the motion of the ball releases those muscles from the point of attachment all along their length. The rolling sets off additional stimulations, creating a chain reaction.

She usually starts her instruction by asking students to sit on the ball, then roll it forward and back along the thigh. This stimulates the lowest part of the pelvis. The pressure of the rolling ball elongates the hamstring muscle and tendon, releasing tension.

"This is not about stretching and feeling the 'burn,'" says Yamuna. "It's about unsticking the parts of the body that have gotten glued together. We figuratively iron them out so that there is space between them again. And this stimulates bones, tendons, circulation, nerve roots, and organ function."

Yamuna pays special attention to the spine, which she considers the key to posture. She asks students to "roll up" each side of the spine. "As you do so," she says, "you lift each vertebra. After all, gravity makes everything drop. In lifting the vertebrae, we get the space back. Again, the rolling stimulates the nerve roots along each vertebra and stimulates organ function, so the body as a whole works better." Better function, of course, translates into better appearance.

Simultaneous Stimulation and Relaxation

The effect is as relaxing as it is stimulating. Says Yamuna: "The rolling also provides a deep relaxation response, so while I like to roll out the spine first thing in the morning to get out any stiffness, it's also a way to unwind and relax and go to sleep."

The entire body feels the benefits of the rolling. Lying facedown and rolling the abdomen from the pubic bone "stimulates all the internal organs," says Yamuna. "It is particularly good for women after childbirth, but it's also great to keep your stomach from sagging. After all, if you sit all day, your stomach muscles drop;

Food Comparison Demonstrations

Each demonstration offers you two choices. The two choices may represent different quantities of food that are calorically equivalent, or foods of similar tastes with radically different calorie counts. In other words, these demonstrations provide graphic evidence of the real calorie cost of many of your favorite foods.

But they show you something else as well. See the icons? They represent different substances in food—some that raise your risk of disease and are bad for you, others that lower your disease risk and/or promote health and are very, very good for you.

Here are the bad-for-you icons. They represent:

Saturated fat and cholesterol	SF ☹
Trans fat	TF ☹
Animal protein	AP ☹
Carcinogens	CA ☹
Refined carbohydrates	RC ☹

And here are the good-for-you icons, representing:

Fiber	F ☺
Phytonutrients	PN ☺
Soy protein	SP ☺
Good fats	GF ☺

Put it all together, and the total picture tells you something important: The kind of eating that is best for weight loss is also best for your health.

Note: Even though fish and shellfish constitute animal proteins, we don't assign them the animal protein icon because the protein they contain is easier on the kidneys and bones. Similarly, even though fish and shellfish contain cholesterol, they are so low in saturated fat that their presence in a demo does not warrant the icon for saturated fat.

Healthy Appetite?

A sizable bowl of Curried Pumpkin Soup is a meal unto itself—and one of the healthiest meals you can eat. It's filled with disease-fighting, health-promoting vegetables, and it has the added benefit of soy protein. Yet its calorie count is only equal to that of this modest morsel of mozzarella, representing the health detriments of animal protein, saturated fat, and cholesterol. If you're hungry for a lot of food, hungry for health, and hungry for a rich, zesty taste, go for the soup.

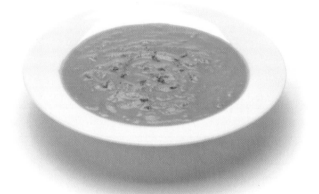

2 cups Curried Pumpkin Soup*   **170 calories**

F   PN   SP

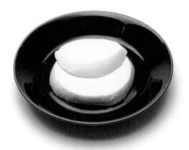

2 oz. mozzarella   **170 calories**

AP   SF   CA

*Recipe given.

Not So Sloppy Joes

Think Sloppy Joes have to be made with beef? Think again. The Sloppy Joe on the top was made with soy-based veggie beef but has a piquant barbecue taste that will make you think it's hot off the skillet. At 110 calories and with lots of health benefits, it's a not-so-sloppy replacement for the Joe on the bottom: 250 calories of animal protein, plus saturated fat and cholesterol of course.

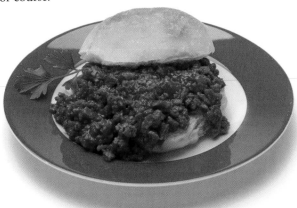

1 cup Vegetarian Sloppy Joes*   **110 calories**

F   PN   SP
😊   😊   😊

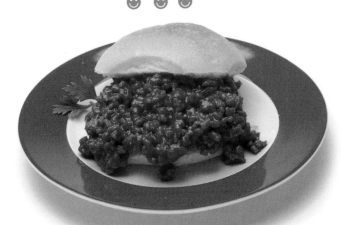

1 cup ground-beef Sloppy Joes   **250 calories**

AP   SF   CA
☹   ☹   ☹

*Recipe given.

Pepper to Taste

If it's pepper and spices you like, try Peppered Sea Bass. It's coated with mustard, sprinkled with peppercorns, then sautéed in oil till it gets that golden brown color. It's a much better protein pick than the steak au poivre below it—and at less than half the calories.

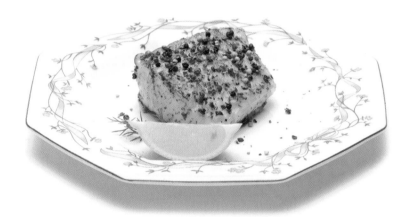

4 oz. Peppered Sea Bass* **170 calories**

GF

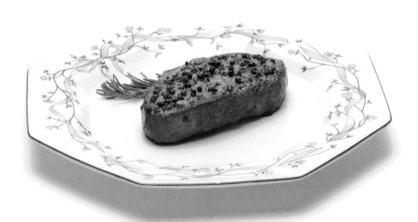

4 oz. steak au poivre **360 calories**

AP SF CA

*Recipe given.

Change Your Chili

The chili on the top is as spicy, as rich, as hearty, and fully as tasty as the chili on the bottom. The difference? The chili on the bottom has meat—and nearly five times as many calories. It also has ingredients that can raise your risk of any number of diseases, while Picture Perfect Chili has ingredients that can lower your risk of those same diseases. Get the taste, but lose the risk and the calories.

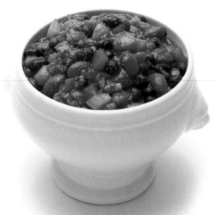

1 cup Picture Perfect Chili*   **150 calories**

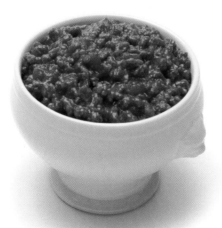

1 cup chili con carne   **530 calories**

*Recipe given.

Taste of Italy

If you like Italian food—and who doesn't?—try Baked Eggplant Casserole with Veggie Ground Beef. It has all the tastes, textures, and health benefits of the Mediterranean style of eating, with one great big added bonus: soy protein. And it has less than half the calories of the meat lasagna on the facing page. Either food makes you think you're in a café on the Via Veneto, but with the eggplant casserole, you raise your chances of living long enough and well enough to get there and really enjoy la dolce vita.

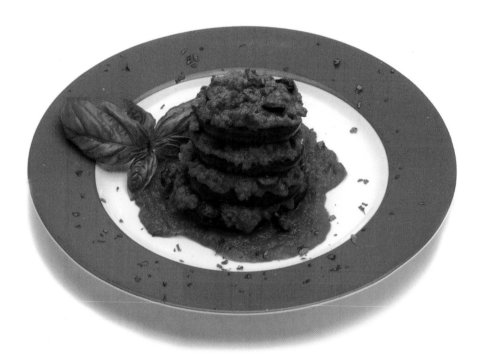

8-oz. serving Baked Eggplant Casserole with Veggie Ground Beef*
145 calories

F PN SP GF

*Recipe given.

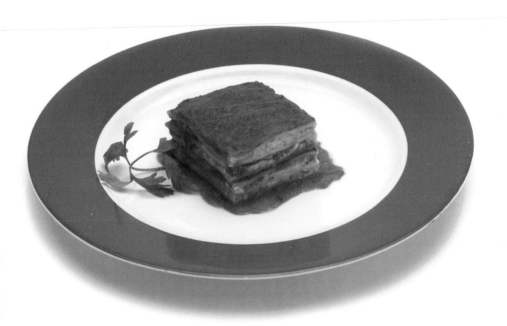

8-oz. serving meat lasagna
380 calories

AP SF CA
☹ ☹ ☹

Eggsactly Right

There are times when only egg salad will do: at a picnic, in your sandwich, on a hot summer day. A cup of regular old egg salad, shown on the bottom, not only costs you 580 calories right now; it may cost you a higher risk of the major killer diseases soon. Try Curried "Egg" Salad, pictured on the top. Filled with spices and textured like regular egg salad, this soy-based dish has only 220 calories—and offers you health benefits you cannot measure.

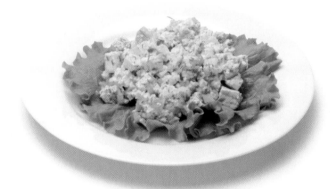

1 cup Curried "Egg" Salad*   **220 calories**

GF   PN   SP

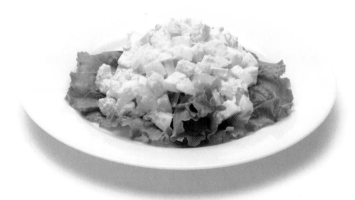

1 cup regular egg salad   **580 calories**

SF

*Recipe given.

Peanut Butter? Are You Kidding?

Well known as one of the good fats, especially if you use natural peanut butter, it is also notorious for its calorie count. Peanut Butter Delight lets you enjoy the taste of peanut butter without a high calorie count—and without the trans fat that raises your risk of disease. So stick with this dessert—and enjoy it!

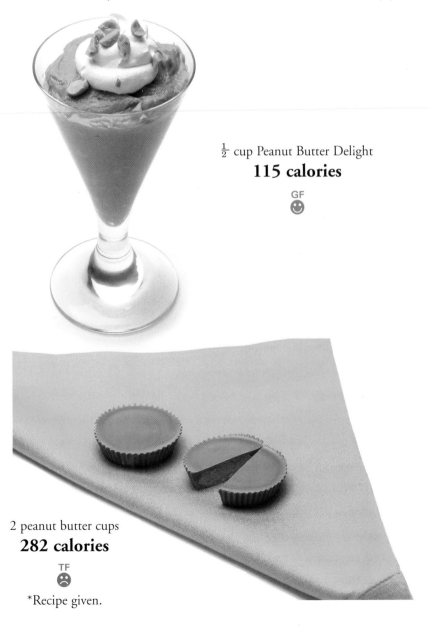

$\frac{1}{2}$ cup Peanut Butter Delight
115 calories

GF
☺

2 peanut butter cups
282 calories

TF
☹

*Recipe given.

Pearing Up

You won't easily find a dessert as elegant or festive as Poached Pears with Sherry—fit for an aristocrat's table. That the dish is also good for you, packed with fiber and phytonutrients, makes it even richer. If you took your pears in tart form and wanted an equal calorie count, you would get only this small piece shown on the facing page—and you'd be taking in unhealthy saturated fat as well.

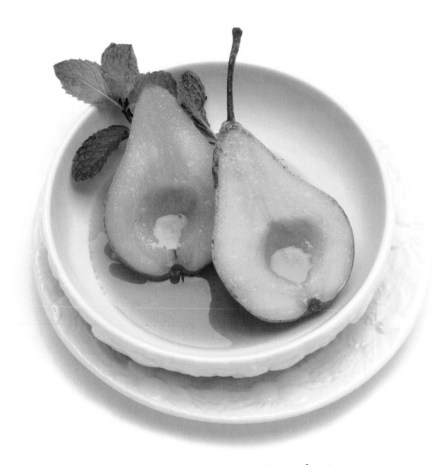

Poached Pears with Sherry*   **100 calories**

F   PN

*Recipe given.

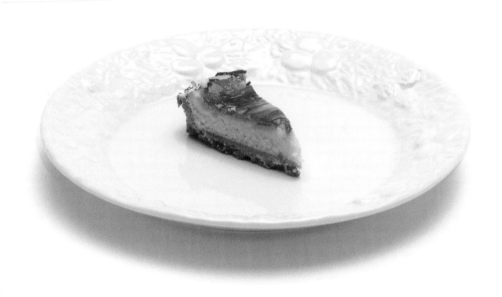

$\frac{1}{4}$ serving pear tart
100 calories

SF   RC

Cold Snap

A great snack or dessert, Ginger-Fruit Yogurt combines the sweetness of fruit, the cool of yogurt, and the snap of ginger in a taste fest that is also chock-full of health benefits. Yet all that comes in at fewer calories than a cup of yogurt from the supermarket (containing more health detriments than you were aware of).

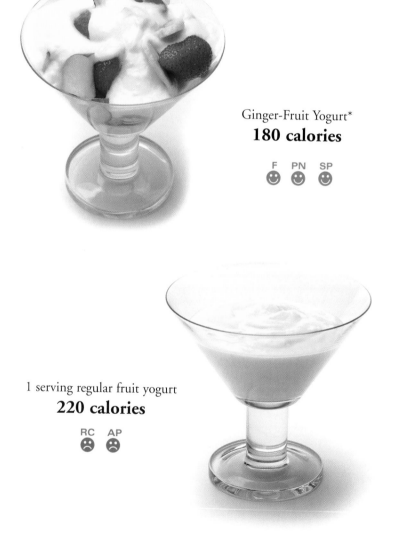

Ginger-Fruit Yogurt*
180 calories

F PN SP
😊 😊 😊

1 serving regular fruit yogurt
220 calories

RC AP
☹️ ☹️

*Recipe given.

Cheesecake Choice

How much cheesecake do you like? It takes two servings of the Individual No-Bake Cheesecakes, shown on the top, to equal the calorie count of that one small cheesecake pictured below. And where the regular cheesecake is filled with substances that can harm your health, the no-bake version boasts things that benefit your health—and lower your risk of disease. As for the taste of the no-bake, it's choice.

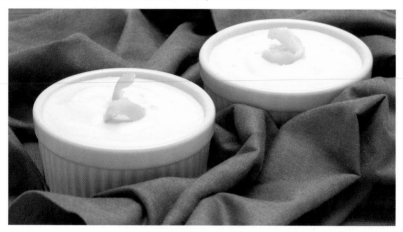

2 servings Individual No-Bake Cheesecakes*   **370 calories**

PN SP GF

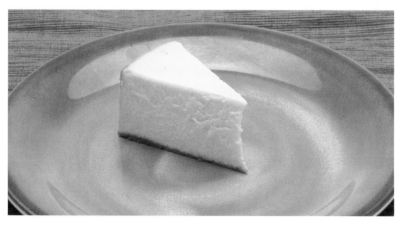

1 serving regular cheesecake   **370 calories**

RC SF CA

*Recipe given.

Pie Pales Next to Pudding

When you crave the taste of pumpkin, get it in luscious Orange and Spice Pumpkin Pudding instead of in conventional pumpkin pie. The pie has five times the calorie count of the pudding and is filled with saturated fat and cholesterol, trans fat, and refined carbs, while the pudding offers healthful fiber and phytonutrients. Pudding is the pick, not pie.

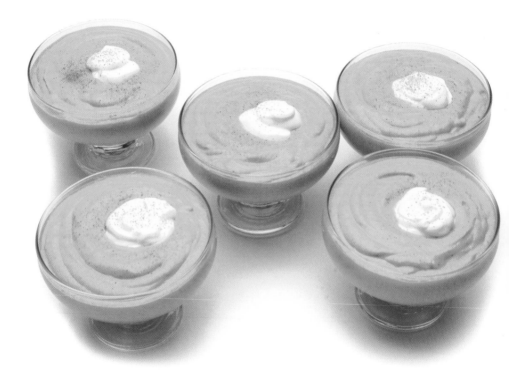

5 servings Orange and Spice Pumpkin Pudding*

325 calories

F   PN

*Recipe given.

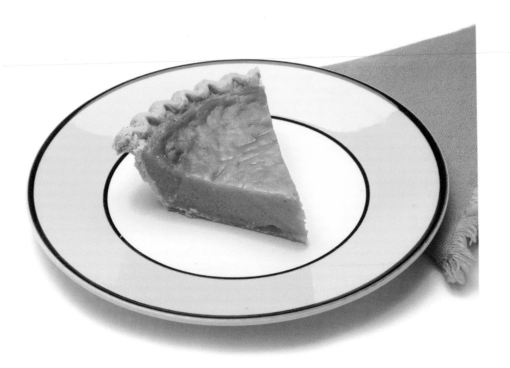

1 serving pumpkin pie
325 calories

TF SF CA RC

Time for Dessert

It's time for dessert, and here are your choices:

On the bottom, a cup of super-premium ice cream, undoubtedly tasty and costing you 600 calories—so put it on your every-now-and-again list.

On top, a fruit cup containing sorbet, whipped topping, and exquisite dark chocolate curls for a grand total of 250 calories. Unseen ingredients here are health-promoting fiber and phytonutrients. If it's time for health and weight loss, it's time for this dessert.

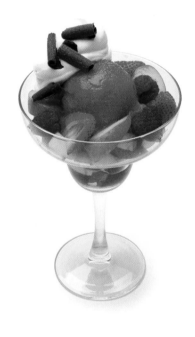

Fruit cup
250 calories

F   PN   RC

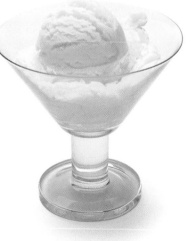

1 cup super-premium ice cream
600 calories

RC   SF   CA

Bread for Breakfast

The buttered bagel is a New York classic, and it adds up to some 640 calories empty of nutrients and packed with saturated fat and cholesterol. Instead, go for two slices of whole-wheat toast, slap on some peanut butter, and add in a cup of fruit, and you're still nowhere near the bagel's calorie count.

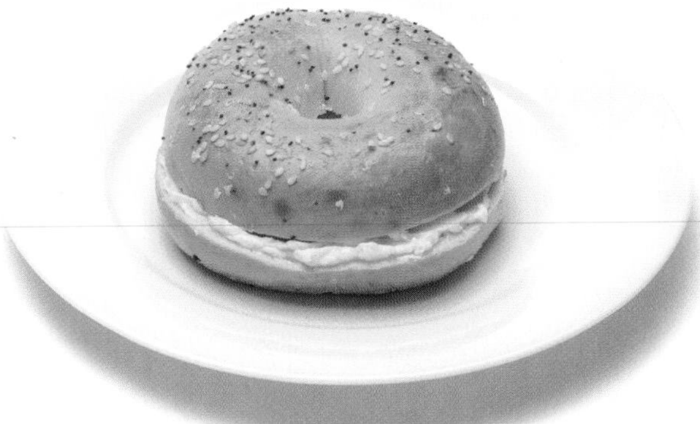

1 5-oz. bagel, 400 calories, + 2 Tbsp. butter, 240 calories = **640 calories**

RC SF

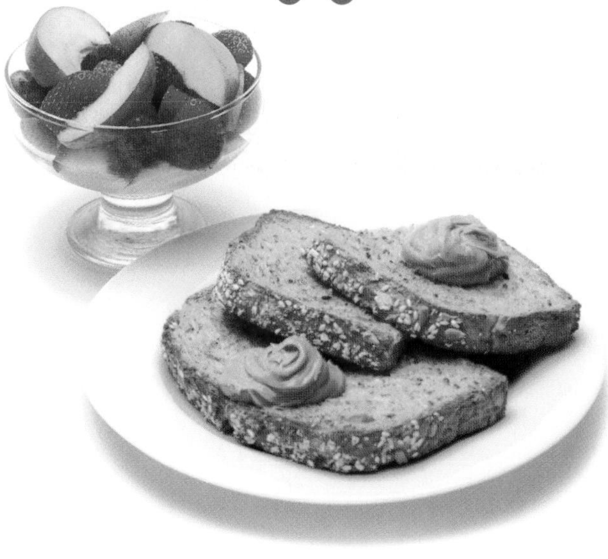

2 slices of whole-wheat toast, 140 calories, + 2 Tbsp. peanut butter, 180 calories, + 1 cup of fruit, 50 calories = **370 calories**

F PN GF

Getting Whet

Appetizers are meant simply to whet your appetite for the meal to come, but you can choose among them so that you save most of your calories for the imminent dinner. Below is a platter of mini-quiches and pigs in a blanket; the quiches alone are 300 calories, and the pigs in a blanket add another 270 for a grand total of 570 calories. Or, choose the refreshing shrimp cocktail in cocktail sauce for 140 calories, yummy grilled mushrooms—a sensational health bonus—costing only 50 calories for all six, and this platter of cucumber slices and crabmeat for 200 calories. The total for this entire collection of appetizers is a mere 390 calories—plus health-giving benefits.

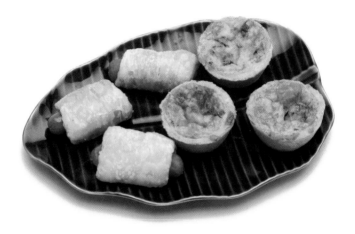

3 mini-quiches and 3 pigs in a blanket

570 calories

AP SF CA TF

☹ ☹ ☹ ☹

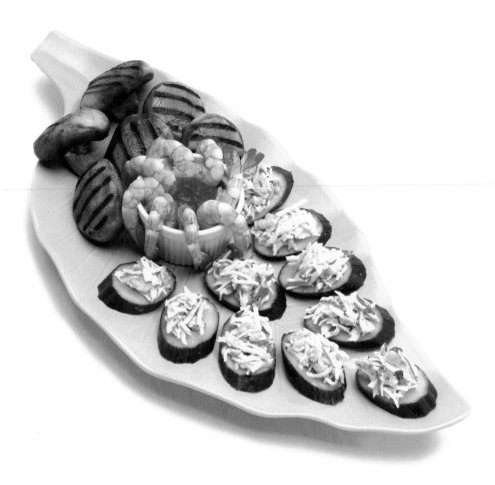

4 oz. shrimp with cocktail sauce + 6 mushrooms grilled with
black bean sauce + 10 cucumber slices with crabmeat salad

390 calories

F   PN

Fat Chance

Sure, this *low-carb* ice cream sounds like it's good for you—till you take a look at the amount of saturated fat it contains, represented here by these five pats of butter. As for calorie count, you could eat ten low-calorie Fudgsicles for the same 300 calories—not that anyone should eat that many Fudgsicles in one sitting. So save the fat and the calories, and take a chance on a low-calorie Fudgsicle when you want something sweet and creamy for dessert.

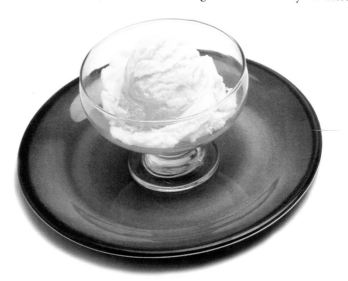

1 cup low-carb ice cream   **300 calories**

SF   CA

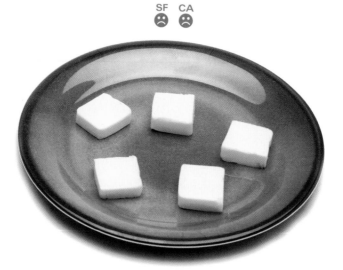

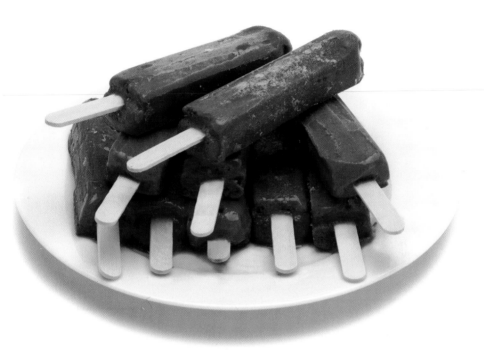

10 Low-Calorie Fudgsicles
300 calories

Low-Carb Salads

This benign-looking chef's salad, with turkey, cheese, and blue cheese dressing, is low in carbs but weighs in at 890 calories and is filled with animal protein, saturated fat and cholesterol, and carcinogens. Take the salad on the facing page instead. At 650 calories, it's a better weight-loss choice, and its plentiful phytonutrients, fiber, and good fat make it a filling bowl of health as well.

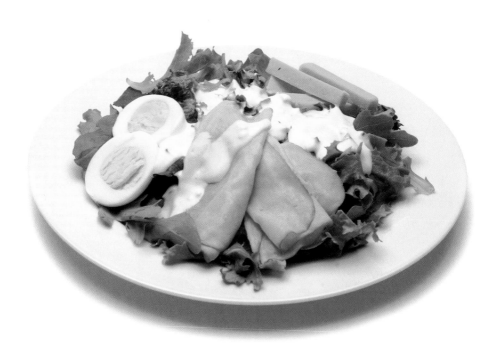

Chef's salad:
2 cups of greens, 3 oz. turkey, 3 oz. cheese, 1 egg,
4 Tbsp. blue cheese dressing

890 calories

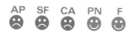

AP   SF   CA   PN   F

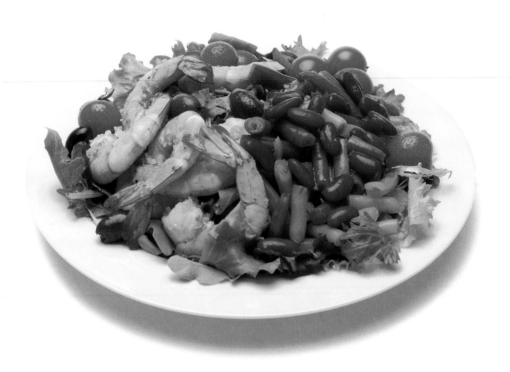

Low-carb salad:
2 cups of greens, 3 oz. shrimp, 1 cup three-bean salad,
6 olives, 6–8 cherry tomatoes, 4 Tbsp. Italian dressing
650 calories

F   PN   GF

Kebabs

It looks pretty simple, but this beef kebab is a complex package of calories, saturated fat, cholesterol, carcinogens, and animal protein. Instead, try this scallop-and-mushroom kebab with a tasty Thai peanut sauce—low in calories and with phytonutrients.

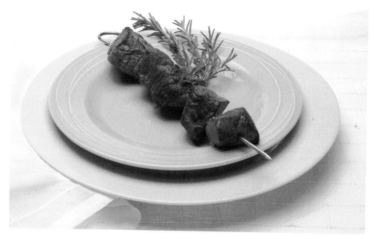

5 oz. beef kebab **560 calories**

AP   SF   CA

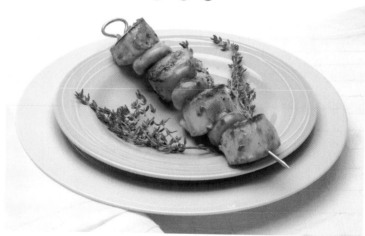

4 oz. scallops, 120 calories, + 4 oz. mushrooms, 15 calories, + 2 Tbsp. Thai peanut sauce, 15 calories = **150 calories**

PN   GF

Fruitful Eating

This plate of sweetened dried fruit may offer you some phytonutrients, but you pay a high price in refined carbohydrates. You don't solve the problem by going for a salty taste; these pretzels, for the same calorie count, are also loaded with refined carbs. Your best bet is the unsweetened dried fruit—filled with fiber and phytonutrients, with not a single refined carb in sight.

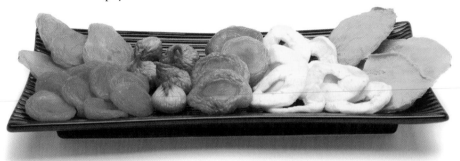

8 dried apricot halves, 64 calories, 8 dried apple slices, 60 calories
3 dried pear halves, 90 calories, 4 dried peach halves, 66 calories
5 dried figs, 150 calories, 3 dried mango slices, 60 calories

total **490 calories**

F   PN

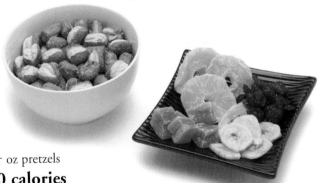

$7\frac{1}{2}$ oz pretzels
810 calories

RC

2 oz dried papaya, 180 calories
2 oz dried pineapple slices, 190 calories
2 oz dried cranberries, 180 calories
2 oz banana chips, 260 calories

total **810 calories**

F   PN   RC

Barbecue Battle

At the barbecue over at the Joneses', you can get a small plate with a burger, a few morsels of sausage, and half a cup of macaroni salad—not to mention a heap of disease-promoting substances. But it's the Joneses who aren't keeping up. Next door at the Smiths', just look at the cornucopia that fills up the jumbo platter they give you: a skewer of shrimp and red peppers, burger and sausage veggie-style, corn on the cob, a healthy portion of zucchini and yellow squash, and a grilled red onion—with all the phytonutrient power, filling fiber, and soy protein those foods represent. And when you finish all that, come back for the watermelon—for even more fiber power. Total calorie count—if you can eat all that food: the same 560 calories.

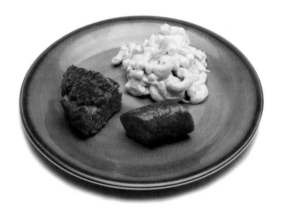

2 oz. burger + 2 oz. sausage + $\frac{1}{2}$ cup macaroni salad
560 calories

AP SF CA RC
☹   ☹   ☹   ☹

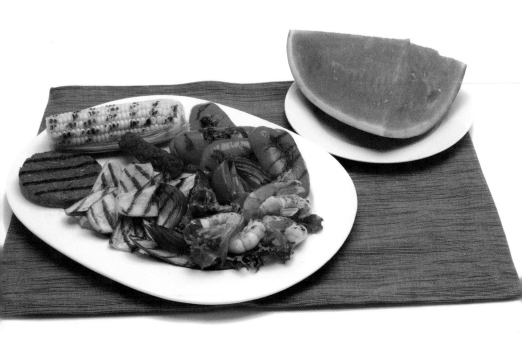

2 oz. shrimp and red peppers + 2 oz. veggie burger + 2 oz. veggie sausage, corn on the cob, grilled zucchini and yellow squash, grilled red onion, 1 ½ lbs. watermelon

560 calories

F   PN   SP

We recommend all of the low-carb food products pictured here. All are good sources of protein, fiber, and/or good fat. You will find here a sample of most of the low-carb products called for in the Three-Day Healthy Low-Carb Blitz.

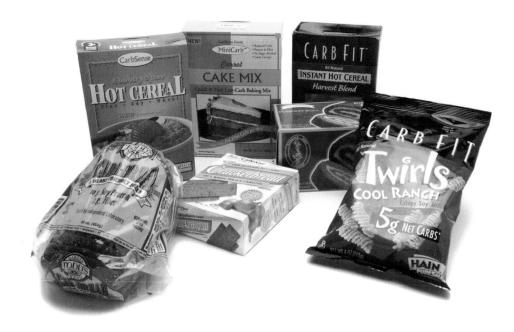

Here is a sampling of some of the soy products we recommend. Look for them among the many soy products available today in your supermarket.

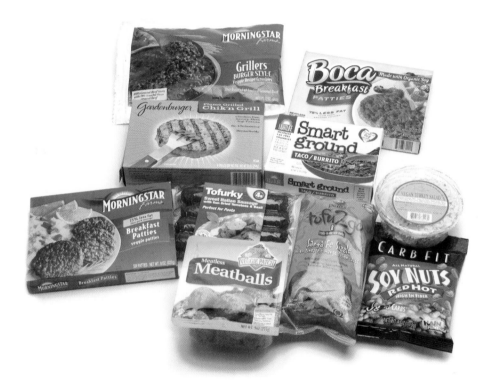

A Day in the Life...
of Three Eating Plans

Dinner and dessert or snack on the Atkins diet, on the South Beach diet, and from the Picture Perfect Pyramid. Three pictures are worth thousands of word…

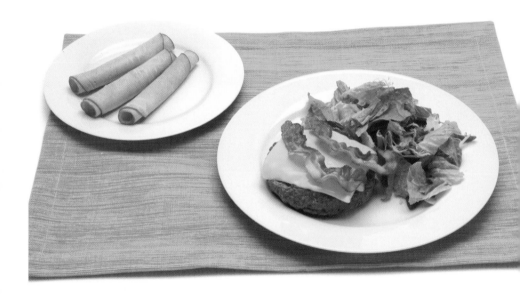

Atkins
Dinner: A large bacon cheeseburger, small green salad
Snack: sliced ham

CA   SF   AP   PN

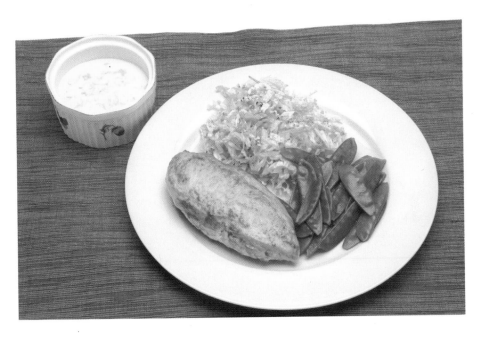

South Beach
Dinner: Gingered Chicken Breast, steamed snow peas, Oriental Cabbage salad
Dessert: Almond Ricotta Creme

AP CA PN F

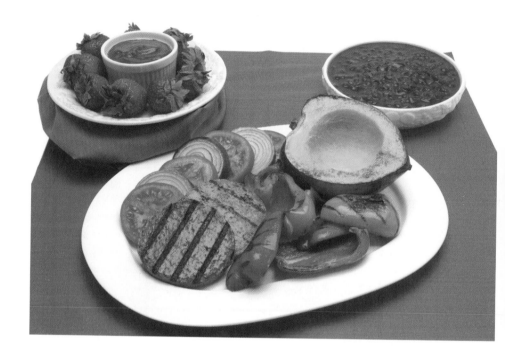

Picture Perfect
Dinner: Black bean soup, veggie burger, grilled mixed peppers,
acorn squash, sliced onions and tomato
Dessert: strawberries with almond-mocha dip*

*Recipe given.

when you lift them, they perk up and hold you up. So we roll the core muscles that hold you up. This also gets rid of lower back pain."

Yamuna has developed routines for every part of the body, including legs, chest, shoulders, and especially the feet. "There is nothing in our culture about taking care of feet," she notes, "yet nothing is more essential for mobility. If you keep your feet healthy, you will walk better—on flats or six-inch heels. Your feet won't hurt, your ankles won't collapse." So she has developed special half-spheres for improving foot function and fitness.

It is all about "liberating the body. Where the body is stuck, where it's not supporting you, where you can't move freely, you must give it room and space to function. People will tell you that stiffness as you age is something you just have to live with."

Yamuna has proven that's simply not true. Your muscles don't have to become stiff, nor do you need to become gradually more immobilized. You can roll it out.

"You don't have to accept limitations on your mobility and on feeling good," she remarks. "Release your body, let go of all the tensions in your body. That's how you'll live better and longer."

See the demonstration on the DVD.

PILATES MOVEMENT
Ron Fletcher

"I call the work movement, not exercise," says Ron Fletcher, creator of the Pilates-based Ron Fletcher Work. In this program, Fletcher combines Pilates and dance techniques with his own system of percussive breathing.

"This is about teaching the body how to move with a certain

amount of grace and assurance and presence," says Fletcher. "Exercise, as people understand the word, does not involve the head, the spirit, or deep gratitude for body. What I teach is a way to heighten our entire sense of being, a way to develop true body awareness, to communicate with the body and become aware of all the parts of it, understanding how magnificently they're all put together. When we do, we feel good about ourselves—and everything works better and looks better."

Fletcher has been perfecting the work for decades. A Missouri native, he trained with the visionary choreographer Martha Graham in the 1940s. He later studied with another visionary, Joseph Pilates, and his wife, Clara.

According to Fletcher, both Graham and Pilates were really working along the same lines—one in the area of dance, the other in fitness. Both started by finding the body's center, "the actual center deep in the core of the body, right down by the pubic bone, where everything connects," says Fletcher.

Though Graham and Pilates have clearly influenced Fletcher, his own program is unique. Fletcher's first career was as a professional choreographer and dancer. It was only after he dropped out of show business that he started doing Pilates training. As he learned the system's precise movements based on control and form, he found himself gaining flexibility and strength even beyond what he had known as a dancer. After a year, he opened his own Pilates-based studio in Beverly Hills, where he catered to the cream of Hollywood stardom.

Moving "with awareness from the center," says Fletcher, "builds a girdle of strength all around the body. That is where your power is." When you have hold of your center, when you control the body's power, the entire structure is supported, and you can move freely.

The Body's Inner Architecture

An appreciation for body structure is essential in the Fletcher program. "Being on-center means you have an awareness of the inner architecture of the body," Fletcher explains, "of how it's working: the bones, the way the muscles gather around the bones, then the skin around the muscle. You know, it's like a building. If the first floor is not properly balanced, the second floor will be off-kilter, and the third floor will really tilt."

When we feel pain, Fletcher explains, it's because our bodies are off center. It shows. "The body naturally pulls away from the pain. You push off the wrong way and constantly try to adjust, and you simply lose the center."

To prevent this, Fletcher has people "go right back to the foundation." Place the feet properly. Align the leg muscles right up to the center.

The center is "where the power and glory are," says Fletcher. "You must get hold of it and understand it. And then the body will lift. You will create more space between your lower rib and hip bone, and the low belly muscles will pull back toward the spine to protect it and make it stronger. Then the spine will straighten, the stomach will straighten, the pelvis will stop tilting backward, and you will hold yourself in a nice long line from the tailbone all the way up, bringing the head back."

Right away, this process of finding the center will improve your appearance. But there's more. "It's not just that you'll gain the cosmetic benefits of a more shapely, compact body in which to stand or move, but everything—all the organs—will be held nicely in their correct places, and the body will work more efficiently. Then you can reach for the sky and open your chest and present yourself. You can truly fill your space, living more completely because you're living gratefully and proudly within this divine mechanism, the body, this fantastic mechanism that most people don't take advantage of."

Nurturing the Divine Mechanism

Fletcher also has developed his own percussive breathing techniques, in which the air is inhaled sharply and rhythmically and exhaled through pursed lips, enhancing the efficiency of the exchange of oxygen and carbon dioxide between the lungs and the bloodstream.

The work was always about more than just moving well or breathing efficiently, however. It was always about "feeling good about ourselves through using our body correctly and breathing well. Everything improves when we do: bones, musculature, skin, hair, eyes as our cells are vitalized. All our senses are enhanced, and it shows everywhere because we're more totally alive."

Think of children, Fletcher urges. "They are born dancers. They fly around and fling their arms freely and easily. It is pure celebratory movement. But as we grow up, we develop all our little fears. We say 'Oh, I can't do that,' and that idea gets stuck in our heads. What I'm aiming for in the work is to get back to the wonder of using our bodies correctly, of not apologizing for being in our space but rather of gratefully realizing all the potential of this divine mechanism we were given to live in. Every body is beautiful, and I want everyone to realize all the potential of their own body, mind, breath, and spirit."

There's nothing wrong with hard physical activity, but Fletcher has words of advice for people who do strenuous exercise. "Running is good," he says, "but it depends how you run. Running in some sloppy old way is not the best thing to do. It's the specificity with which we use our bodies that's important. That doesn't mean there aren't times when we just flop and let go, but we must nurture the body, explore how wondrously it works, and build on the divine gift of the body."

It is all of a piece. To nurture this "divine mechanism," you must not just move well and breathe well but choose carefully what you take into the body, keep it free from stress, take care of it in every way. All of it, says Fletcher, shows "that we really are worthy of ourselves. Standing up straight, eating well, moving with grace, lengthening our muscles and soft tissues, breathing correctly, letting our bodies speak with eloquence: it all is a matter of being totally alive. The point is to honor the body and get in touch with it, to feel it, and be present in it. And that's a joy."

See the demonstration on the DVD.

TAI CHI
Lawrence Tan

"An ordinary person can unleash extraordinary power by learning how to unify mind, body, and spirit," says martial arts grand master Lawrence Tan. His words express the core of the teachings of tai chi.

Tai chi, says Tan, "is a way of taking care of yourself through movement. By controlling the mind, body, and spirit, you can be healthier and happier and can increase your life span."

Tan, a Chinese-American, first became enamored of the ancient

Chinese martial arts in high school. After studying karate, judo, and kung fu, he then began learning the gentler discipline of tai chi. All the martial arts, he notes, are what he calls "multidimensional."

In undertaking tai chi training, a person is not only dealing with physical fitness, but also with the mind "in a spiritual dimension." Developed by ancient warrior-monks as a means of self-defense, the martial arts combined military movement with artistic discipline. The idea, says Tan, was "power concealed in elegance." That remains the core of martial arts training.

Although the philosophy behind this can take years of study to understand fully, it derives from a worldview that can be explained fairly simply. Think of the world as having three planes—the spiritual plane of the heavens above, the physical plane of the earth below, and the plane of reason represented by human beings in between heaven and earth.

"If these forces are not aligned, the result is conflict, confusion, and chaos," Tan explains. But by learning how to align them, "we can maximize our power and achieve peace and harmony." That is why a 98-pound woman who is superbly trained in martial arts really can toss a 200-pound male athlete over her shoulder.

Power Through Pliability

The alignment of the natural order involves more than power. "We can be healthier and less stressed if we can live in harmony with these natural laws," Tan says. "If rain is coming, instead of fighting it, we must just accept it and do what is appropriate."

That pliability is at the heart of tai chi. Its practitioners sometimes liken themselves to bamboo—strong yet pliable. The bamboo plant, they say, allows itself to bend in the face of a stiff wind; that is why it survives. Tai chi therefore includes ways of moving "that focus on being soft, flowing, and able to flex along with the changes in life and nature." Moreover, every movement of tai chi practice has a hidden meaning, says Tan. Moving your hand in a certain way, for example, "will work on certain points to increase blood flow and raise your energy level throughout the body."

Moving Meditation

Classic tai chi consists of a course of slow-motion movements that teach the mind to be focused and aware. Anyone who has ever visited China—or perhaps a Chinese neighborhood in the United States—has probably seen the early-morning practitioners of tai chi performing their slow, elegant movements, hands and bodies carving the air with stately precision.

The term for this practice is "moving meditation." Its purpose is definitely "not just physical," Tan says. "It is about how to control the emotions and focus and clear the mind." The original idea behind this mind work is that "the more mentally aware you are in combat, the more effective you will be. Precisely because you know how to move in a relaxed way, when you do need to move fast, you will do it with more power."

But this slow and graceful practice can take time—which may be why many of those early-morning tai chi practitioners are elderly, retired folks. For those who cannot spend hours practicing the movements, *Tan has devised a universal form of tai chi–based wellness exercises that offer the same benefits in less time.*

"Because this moving meditation is of great value for the average person's health, I took the essence of the movements and created a short form that people can do any time, any place. *It is a*

*whole cycle of movements with a beginning, middle, and end,
but it takes only from a minute to five minutes to do.*"

With Tan's universal form of tai chi, you still move the body,
concentrate the mind, and breathe as in classic tai chi, and you still
gain the benefits of unifying those three aspects: "a centered, calm
state of mind and being."

The value of the universal form, Tan claims, is that "you're not
going to sleep, but you're resting the body. The mind is aware but
calm and clear so that you can, in fact, reach peak performance." It
is a form of exercise that is "so valuable as we age because unlike
other forms of activity that put stress on the heart, this works on
the circulatory and respiratory systems, oxygenating the body. And
it does so without any stress on the heart or musculature. In fact,
it helps develop muscularity and strength."

See the demonstration on the DVD.

CORE FUSION
Fred DeVito

It is "endlessly challenging," in the words of creator Fred
DeVito, and it leaves you "calm, relaxed, focused, but with muscles
tingling when you walk out of the room."

Core Fusion, as its name implies, is the ultimate merging of
different exercise techniques and philosophies to shape the body
and provide what DeVito calls "a transformational mind-body
fitness experience."

Body Shaping, Conditioning, Balance

Developed in 2002 at the New York headquarters of the Exhale Mindbodyspa by husband-and-wife team Fred DeVito and Elisabeth Halfpapp, Core Fusion combines yoga, Pilates, orthopedic exercises, and core conditioning. DeVito says Core Fusion provides "body shaping for people who need to tone, sports conditioning for weekend athletic warriors, and a form of progressive rehabilitation for people who have been injured and who need balance in their body."

The hour-long Core Fusion workout—or its half-hour "express" version—focuses on flexibility and strength. So if you've become too tight, perhaps from lifting heavy weights, or if you're loose-limbed and lack strength through a range of motion, Core Fusion brings you back into balance.

In addition, a meditative element of the Core Fusion program offers physical relaxation and a reenergizing of the spirit. The results are a well-toned body and a feeling of what DeVito calls "calm energy."

Hard Work

Professional trainers with backgrounds in physical education, dance, and a range of exercise techniques, DeVito and Halfpapp began to notice that many of their clients weren't getting the kind of training they needed. Veterans of strenuous gym workouts and adept users of fitness machines, these clients had put in substantial time and effort on weight training and aerobics. But flexibility and core strength were still lacking. With the creation of the Core Fusion program, DeVito and Halfpapp came up with an intensely rigorous program that "works" both body and mind.

"You really need to leave your ego at the door," DeVito says of Exhale's Core Fusion class, "because the session can be humbling. It is hard work."

There are no machines in Core Fusion. The body itself provides resistance, as the individual moves efficiently at an interval-training pace while focusing intently on form and positioning to produce fast results.

Each session starts with a warm-up, then moves to exercises aimed at strengthening the lower body and increasing its flexibility. Then on to core conditioning for abdominal strength and lower-back flexibility. All this is followed by Savasana, the meditative yoga relaxation pose that reenergizes the spirit. Each session concludes with a final series of stretches for cooldown and balance.

It is a demanding session, requiring a lot of energy. "It doesn't matter how often or how long you've been doing it; it's endlessly challenging," observes DeVito. "It is like playing a musical instrument. You can become very competent, but you can still find music that challenges you. With Core Fusion, you're working with your body in space—there is no equipment—so there are always different variables you can tweak. You can increase the intensity or the duration, or you can challenge the posture itself by making it more complicated. So you can always add to the mix to raise the level of the challenge. No matter how strong or how flexible you become, you can always add another degree."

A Good Break

Core Fusion work is revitalizing and reenergizing in every way. With the physical effort, you get what DeVito calls "tingling muscles." But to get the most out of a session requires full commitment. "When you come into the room," says DeVito, "you must be ready to undergo one hour of uninterrupted concentration, so it's a good mental break as well as a physical one." And when you leave, you take with you both the tingling sensation in your body and the calm energy in your mind—a fusion of mind-body results following this fusion of mind-body activities.

See the demonstration on the DVD.

PERSONAL TRAINING
Heather Raymond

"Find your path," says fitness professional Heather Raymond. "And when you do," she adds, "challenge your limit."

Raymond, who began teaching aerobics at age fifteen, is licensed as both a personal trainer and a massage therapist. She meets her private clients wherever they are most comfortable—at home, at the gym, in a park—and works with the client to "bring to them whatever they need for their particular goal."

That personal fitness goal is the starting point, says Raymond. "I ask clients: 'What do you want to get out of this? What excites you?' If someone is into golf, then maybe we start with a program that will offer a tangible improvement in golf. Maybe it's that someone has had a health scare, or that their high school reunion is coming up, or they've noticed they're stiff in the morning, or just that they want to look hot. Then we create a program that's very specific to the individual and that shows respect for the person's particular level of fitness."

Be the Boss of Your Own Story

It's important, says Raymond, to "take it in steps. Each time a person achieves something tangible, they will automatically set the bar higher for themselves, and they will also want to make other improvements in their health and lifestyle. If a client learns that she can lift weights, then she wants to quit smoking, then to eat more healthfully, then to lift more weights. And so on. And that is how people build their level of fitness."

Fitness Raymond defines as "a state of high-level homeostasis. When all your body functions work properly and at a high level, when you are achieving and maintaining a high level of health, that is fitness."

Even the first steps toward fitness—the most basic exercise programs—"enhance your general health. When you are exercising, you are taking active control of your health, and that improves your overall quality of life.

"This is terribly important psychologically, too," Raymond continues. "Exercise lifts you above your daily scenario. You feel better about where you are and what you can do. In a world where so much is left to chance, exercise gives you a feeling of empowerment over your body's shape and your appearance. You become the boss of your own story."

That is why Heather Raymond draws upon all forms of exercise in helping her clients find their path. Yoga, Pilates, weight training, cardiovascular workouts, stretching, lifestyle exercise: she uses them all—and more—to create each client's pathway to the goal they have set.

Yet if there's one form of exercise that seems to summarize Raymond's ideas about exercise, it is perhaps weight training. First, the benefits of weight training dramatically illustrate the benefits of exercise in general. "You build muscle and look fit," Raymond says simply. "Every pound of muscle you put on your body allows you to eat 250 more calories—because you are burning calories and losing fat as you build muscle. Your metabolism is stronger, your clothes fit better, your confidence rises as your strength rises, and you are empowered—whether it is because you can now carry your own suitcase or because you can press one hundred pounds. The kind of strengthening you get from weight training also has psychological benefits—it's a big stress fighter—and can improve numerous medical conditions."

Lift Weights—and Raise Your Confidence

Press, curl, squat, lunge, lift, hold—and raise your self-esteem and sense of empowerment. Whatever your age, the stronger you are, the more energetic you feel. The more energetic you feel, you more you do. The more you do, the greater your confidence.

And the confidence that comes from greater strength can help fight depression. A study of moderately depressed older individuals found that those assigned to a supervised weight-training program three times a week enjoyed a remarkable reduction in depression, dramatic improvement in self-confidence levels—and a much better night's sleep.

But beyond the physical and psychological benefits, weight training is a form of exercise in which people can almost literally see themselves challenge their limits. "You up the ante every time you work out," Raymond explains. "I always ask my clients for one more pound of weight or one more repetition. So they are always going to the edge of what the body can do, then taking one gentle step more. Always challenge your limit. If you think your limit is eight reps, do eight more. And then you find that you can. If you think you can do ten push-ups, you can probably do twenty.

"Halfway there," she concedes, "you probably will start fearing that you're not going to make it. You'll start feeling pain. But then you pull from within to go one step further—one more rep, one more push-up—and that is how you feel the success as you go."

For Raymond, this isn't only a fact of weight-training progress; it is also a metaphor for any challenge. "In the middle stages of the path," she says, "you feel pain, limitations, rejection. The important thing is to understand that that is normal. It's a normal stage on the path. It is on the way to success."

The term of art in weight training is to "go to failure." Explains Raymond: "It means that you exhaust the muscle's power without deviating from form. When you do push-ups to failure, for example, it means you keep going until you absolutely cannot do another push-up on form, until your muscle is shaking and you cannot comfortably or without injury do another one. So when we say go to failure, we mean keep going, stay with the proper form, and just keep doing one more until you simply cannot."

It is in going to failure, says Raymond, that "you get to success. In a very real sense, success is achieved through failure." In Raymond's view, always adding one more—always pushing toward failure—is precisely what advances the positive. No wonder her favorite quote is that line attributed to Gandhi: "Be the change you want to see"—and challenge your limit to do so.

"The principle is to push," she says, "to reach inside yourself and trust that you can go beyond where you think you are." You don't do it by chatting as you do a few reps, or by racing through a workout. In fact, the slower the better—first, because it is safer, and second, because going slowly forces you to concentrate, lets you focus on what you're doing, enables you to see where you are weak and where you are strong. "While you're working," Raymond urges, "just work. Be there, present in the moment, focusing on your eventual goal."

Change Your Relationship with Food: Lose Weight and Stay Slim

Awareness			
DAY 1	**DAY 2**	**DAY 3**	**DAY 4**
Try something new.	Focus on fish.	Send for soup; hail to whole grains.	Eat your vegetables.

Action						
DAY 5	**DAY 6**	**DAY 7**	**DAY 8**	**DAY 9**	**DAY 10**	**DAY 11**
Strive for the ideal.	Lower your risk of disease.	Lower your calorie intake.	Eat the pyramid way.	Three-Day Healthy Low-Carb Blitz 1	Three-Day Healthy Low-Carb Blitz 2	Three-Day Healthy Low-Carb Blitz 3

Chapter 4

CHANGE YOUR RELATIONSHIP WITH FOOD: LOSE WEIGHT AND STAY SLIM

It's a typical day for a typical family—I'll call them the Joneses—in a typical American town or suburb. The day starts with a Pop-Tart or breakfast bar or a bagel with cream cheese and jelly grabbed in a hurry by Mom, Dad, Johnny, and Susie as they get themselves dressed, ready, and out the door to start their respective days.

For the kids, lunch is a meal of their choice in the school cafeteria. Johnny fills up on meat loaf and mashed potatoes slathered with gravy, washing it all down with a large Coke or two. Susie, who seeks to maintain her still-slim teenager's figure, goes for a Caesar salad with low-fat ranch dressing out of a bottle and plenty of croutons, accompanied by a juice drink. Mom, who is racing from one appointment to the next, picks up a slice of pizza and a cup of coffee. Dad, lunching with a client, is enjoying linguine in cream sauce with garlic bread, and tiramisú for dessert.

What's for Dinner?

The family dinner is neither quite a dinner nor is it taken as a family. The kids, who have both chowed down on fast-food burgers and fries after school, are just home from sports practice and about to go out for the evening—Johnny to study with a friend, Susie to choir rehearsal—so they simply grab a snack. Johnny concocts a sandwich out of packaged ham, packaged cheese, and packaged bread, plus a couple of handfuls of potato chips from the supersized bag, while the health-conscious Susie "dines" on a low-fat muffin covered with honey—and some yogurt-covered pretzels for a treat.

Mom, who is more or less following a popular low-carb diet—this one is said to be "healthy"—is off to the school board meeting, so she just has some leftover cold chicken and a salad, plus a part-skim cheese stick. Meanwhile, she throws a steak on the broiler and a potato in the oven for Dad. He likes melted cheese on his steak, and he won't eat the baked potato without lots of butter and sour cream, but he is handy enough in the kitchen to put together those toppings for himself, so Mom just throws him a kiss as he sits down to his dinner, and she flies out the door.

Sound familiar? Is this anything like your family or your life? If you're at all typical, it probably is.

What Most of Us Eat

Processed food. Packaged snacks. Meals on the run. Thousands of calories a day. Lots of animal foods and minimal fruits and vegetables.

Is it any wonder that our government now tells us that we Americans are quite literally eating ourselves to death? And is it any wonder that Johnny and Susie and their peers constitute the first generation in history destined for a *shorter life span* than that of the preceding generation?

Let me put it as simply and straightforwardly as possible: *The way we eat is killing us*. It is making us fat, and it is setting us up for debilitating and destructive diseases that erode the quality of our lives even as they cut our lives short.

What's wrong with keeping up with the Joneses where eating is concerned? Let's take it a meal at a time.

What's Wrong with That Picture?

While breakfast bars and a quick bagel may be a convenient way to fuel up for the day, they really don't carry the nutritional power of good healthy food. The bagel is not only high in calories, it's also a refined carbohydrate, one from which virtually all nutrients have been removed. The cream cheese on the bagel—and Dad layered it on thickly—is high in saturated fat and cholesterol, well-known contributors to heart disease and stroke. The Pop-Tart and breakfast bar favored by the children take it all a step further: These foods are high in what is called trans fat. It gives the product a longer shelf life and the person eating the product a spike in the "bad," or LDL, cholesterol and a reduction in the "good," or HDL, cholesterol—fertile grounds for heart attack or stroke.

And no one in the family has started the day with that obvious breakfast centerpiece, fruit. Why is this important? Fruits and vegetables in all their color and variety are central to healthy eating, as our mothers told us and as medical science has confirmed time and again.

Fruits and vegetables have fiber, which is essential for health (and also prevents weight gain). Plus, they have vitamins, minerals, and phytonutrients—power-packed substances that fight disease and promote health. And absolutely no one in the Jones family is starting the day armed with these benefits.

Fat Facts		
TYPE OF FAT	EFFECTS*	FOOD SOURCES
Monounsaturated	Lowers total and LDL cholesterol, no effect on HDL cholesterol	Canola oil, peanut oil, olive oil
Omega-3 fatty acids	Lower total and LDL cholesterol, raise HDL cholesterol	Flaxseeds, flax oil, fatty fish, walnuts
Polyunsaturated	Lowers total and LDL cholesterol, may lower HDL cholesterol slightly	Corn oil, safflower oil
Saturated	Raises total and LDL cholesterol	Meat, poultry, dairy, eggs, palm oil
Trans fat	Raises total and LDL cholesterol, may lower HDL cholesterol	Stick margarine, solid shortening, commercially processed crackers, cookies, fried foods
*LDL is the "bad" cholesterol, HDL the "good" cholesterol.		

Out to Lunch

As for lunch, Johnny's probably constitutes the typical American meal—and it's a health minefield. As with far too many meals in our country, animal protein is central to this meal. After all, you might argue, steaks, chops, and burgers are the American way—practically synonymous with American cuisine. And what's wrong with it? Surely there's nothing wrong with protein. It's essential for life, isn't it?

Indeed it is. It builds bone and muscle, repairs tissue, strengthens the immune system, is the basic requirement for growth and maturation. But there are many ways to get needed protein, and getting it from animal foods may be the least healthy way. *It's best to*

eat meat only now and then, and only lean and in moderate amounts.
The most protein should come from beans, other legumes, soy
products, and from fish and shellfish instead.

The reasons for avoiding animal-protein foods are well known.
Many are high in saturated fat and cholesterol. They are also filled with
carcinogens, including hormones, breakdown products of lactose,
insulin-like growth factor, and other substances that increase our
risk of cancer. What's more, these and other substances in animal
protein foods help increase the risk of kidney disease and osteoporosis.
They also escalate our chances of having cardiovascular ailments.
Eaten on a regular basis, animal-protein foods are a bad deal.

In Johnny's case, moreover, since the cafeteria mass-produces
the mashed potatoes from a package, chances are there are no
nutrients left in what otherwise might be a powerful nutritional
vehicle—the potato.

Susie's Caesar salad, by contrast, is a healthy choice—filled
with fiber to help her stay slim and with nutrients that fight
disease. The only problem is, it's midday, and she has yet to eat any
protein at all—particularly unwise in a growing teenager, and
especially a girl. Her bones are still not fully developed—and won't
be, until she reaches her mid-twenties. By skimping on protein,
she's increasing her risk of serious bone loss, osteoporosis, in her
later years.

While the kids' after-school snacks of fast-food burgers constitute
protein, it's again a protein that is high in saturated fat—accompanied
by processed hamburger rolls empty of nutrition and filled with
refined carbs, and by fried potatoes that are high in trans fat.

As for Mom and Dad . . .

Mom's leaner-meat chicken dinner with a side salad may be evidence of her desire to eat more healthfully, but it's also evidence that she is to some extent kidding herself. She's still taking in the unhealthy fats, albeit less of them, and carcinogens. In fact, chicken contains ten times more of a harmful carcinogen called heterocyclic amines than beef.

While the salad gives Mom some good phytonutrients, her low-carb diet restricts her intake of fruits and vegetables. So she is still not getting enough of the health-promoting vitamins, minerals, fiber, and disease fighters present in all plant foods.

Dad's dinner is off-the-charts high in saturated fat, trans fat, cholesterol, and carcinogens. With his calorie-loaded lunch, he's setting himself up for a heart attack before his kids graduate from college—especially since he has managed to get through yet another day without a single fruit or vegetable. He needs the disease-fighting nutrients those foods provide, and he's depriving himself of life-prolonging sustenance while loading up on girth-enhancing calories.

Are the Joneses typical? You bet they are. They, and families like them, eat pretty much like this, day after day. Which is one reason Americans are becoming more and more overweight while they run an ever greater risk of disease and premature death.

A Scolding from Science

Our heavy emphasis on animal protein, our completely inadequate intake of the plant-based spectrum of foods with their disease-fighting powers, and our reliance on the "convenience" of refined and/or processed foods from which the nutrients have

been removed is a way of eating that is resulting in the conditions and diseases that lead to an early death.

How much more data do we need on this subject? Among children, overweight and obesity have become epidemic. *From 1976 to 1980, 6 percent of children ages six to eighteen were overweight. From 1999 to 2000, 15 percent were.* As I write these words, more than 10 percent of preschoolers are overweight, and that number is rising as well.

We are seeing the tragic results in teenagers stricken with Type 2 diabetes—the adult strain of the disease—aand in kids showing early signs of hypertension, high cholesterol, and difficulties of walking and breathing. If they stay on their present course, many will suffer heart attacks when they are in their thirties, if they last till then.

Among adults, the news is not much better. An estimated 60 percent of us are overweight, a third of us are obese. It seems to get worse as we get older. A 2002 study found that the incidence of obesity in those over fifty nearly doubled from 1982 to 1999, growing from 14.4 percent to 26.7 percent.

The consequences of this rampant trend toward overweight and obesity in our population are downright fatal. In 2000, in fact, *obesity officially became the nation's number-two killer,* responsible for some 400,000 American deaths—more than 16 percent of all deaths. That was an increase of 2 percent over the previous decade, so obesity seems well on its way to supplanting tobacco as the nation's most formidable underlying killer.

If you're an *overweight woman,* count on *losing three years* off your life span. If you're an *obese woman*—that is, if you weigh more than 30 percent above your ideal weight—*you will lose more than seven years.* If you're an obese man, say good-bye to nearly six years of life.

These statistics are conclusive: ***Excessive weight can kill***.

But the mortality risk is just for openers. For even when being overweight may not kill you, it can damage your health. Did you know that overweight can adversely affect your respiratory system? Your kidneys? Liver? Sleep patterns? Skin? Immune system? Menstrual cycle? Take a look at the chart below. It summarizes just what being overweight can do to your health. Many of the conditions listed here are killers. All of them, in their own way, are destructive of good living.

If You're Overweight, You're at Risk

The heavier you are, the greater the risk to your health. Certainly, your genetic profile, the number of excess pounds you carry, and your age have a lot to do with just how great your risk is. But the basic fact remains: Being overweight makes you susceptible to numerous diseases and more prone to ill health. What's more, the longer you are overweight, the greater the stress you're inflicting on your entire system, and that in turn makes you even more susceptible. On the next few pages, you'll find just some of the risks you run if you are significantly overweight:

Heart

Increased incidence of irregular heartbeats

Increased blood pressure

Increased resting heart rate

Increased heart size

Increased risk of congestive heart failure

Blood Vessels

Additional blood pathways: 1 pound of fat = 200 miles of additional blood vessels

Inflammation of veins

Increased incidence of arteriosclerosis

Hypertension

Blood

Increased levels of cholesterol, triglycerides, ketones, and insulin

Reduced levels of HDL, or "good," cholesterol

Spinal Column

Lower back problems

Increased risk of ruptured disks

Skeletal System

Restricted mobility

Increased proneness to accidents

(Continued on page 140)

(Continued from page 139)

Orthopedic Problems

Increased incidence of osteoarthritis

Degenerative joint disease

Inflammation of the joints

Muscles

Reduced insulin sensitivity

Impaired glucose metabolism, resulting in diabetic condition

Fat Cells

Increased incidence of diabetes due to increased abdominal fat

Skin

Increased incidence of ulcers

Increased incidence of skin irritations

Increased facial hair

Brain

Increased stroke incidence

Risk of cerebral hemorrhage

Lungs

Increased respiratory distress (sleep apnea)

Inability to exchange gases in lungs

Stomach

Increased incidence of carcinoma

Kidneys

Renal disease

Hypertension

Liver

Increased risk of cancer

Increased incidence of cirrhosis

Pancreas

Increased incidence of carcinoma

Gallbladder

Increased incidence of gallstones

Increased incidence of cancer

Colon

Increased incidence of cancer

Decreased intestinal mobility

Uterus and Ovaries

Increased incidence of fibroids and endometrial cancer

Irregular length of menstrual cycles

Heavy menstrual flow

Reduced reproductive capacity

(Continued on page 142)

Lower Extremities (especially ankles)

Venostasis—blood trapped in extremities by compression of veins

Edema—excessive amount of fluid in body tissues

Immune System

Susceptibility to infections

Psychophysical

Decreased sex drive

Lack of assertiveness

Psychological incapacity

Overall

Increased incidence of hernias

Increased operative risks

Increased organ compression by fat tissue

Domino Effects

It is obvious to doctors and nutritionists that many diseases are related to eating the wrong kinds of food. Now they've found that nutrition and weight-related diseases are also interrelated. In fact, doctors have identified one combination called the ***metabolic syndrome***, or syndrome X. This syndrome includes high blood pressure, obesity, diabetes, and the condition known as dyslipidemia, which is essentially a combination of high total cholesterol; high low-density, or "bad," cholesterol; low high-density, or "good," cholesterol; and high triglycerides.

The conditions of metabolic syndrome are intertwined. All affect the arteries and increase the chance of death from heart attack or stroke. The more conditions of the syndrome a person may suffer, the greater his risk of death from heart attack or stroke. Diabetes patients are two to four times more likely to have heart disease than those without diabetes, and people with hypertension are more likely to become diabetic. And so on. And in all the cases of the syndrome, it is a diet high in animal fats and cholesterol, and low in fruits and vegetables that increases the risk of the metabolic syndrome.

A diet high in animal protein, lean or fat, also greatly increases the risk of osteoporosis, a cruel disease that afflicts between 14 million and 20 million American women, causing frequent bone fractures, pain, and a misshapen body. A Yale University study of hip fracture rates in sixteen countries has confirmed that those countries with the highest consumption of meat, egg, and dairy products have the highest number of bone breaks. The conclusion? Animal protein stimulates bone deterioration and calcium loss.

Advice About Dairy Products

Everyone knows that calcium intake is essential for bone health, but what really counts is not just how much calcium you take in but how much the body retains. The old saw about milk being good for bone health turns out not be true—certainly not where the risk of osteoporosis is concerned: The famous Harvard Nurses' Health Study found that nurses with the highest calcium intake from milk and other dairy products suffered more hip fractures than those who drank the least milk. The reason? High levels of animal protein in the diet leach calcium from the bones.

In fact, one of the most effective dietary factors for bone health is soy. Most soy foods are superb sources of calcium, decrease calcium loss, and may even directly inhibit bone dissolution. Other good calcium foods are the dark green leafy vegetables, nuts, beans, dried figs, and tahini.

Get a New Food Relationship

There is good news: By changing our way of eating, we can change the conditions that can lead to disease. Fortunately, the same kind of healthful eating that enables us to fight debilitating disease is the exact same eating plan that can help us lose pounds and maintain an ideal weight. Change your relationship with food, and you can fight a two-pronged war for longevity: through weight loss and through lowering the risk of disease.

That is precisely what the next eleven days are all about.

But you can't change your food relationship by dieting. For one thing, every study done on the subject reaches the same sad conclusion: People who lose weight on a diet *regain* it; in fact, fully 95 percent of them gain back even more weight than they lost. Why?

Physiologically, the research shows that the metabolic adaptations that take place during a weight-loss diet actually predispose the dieter to regain the weight. The fact is that the human body guards stored fat as a protection against starvation. Deliberately restricting food intake, which is exactly what happens on a diet, prompts the body to lower the dieter's metabolic rate. Once the diet is over and the dieter goes back to normal eating, the less efficient metabolism burns fewer calories.

The Dangers of Yo-yo-ing

There is also evidence that repeated weight loss and gain, called yo-yo dieting, makes it more difficult to lose weight on each succeeding diet. Time after time of adjusting to a lower calorie intake and a slowed metabolic rate simply takes its toll; the body can no longer bounce back from diet to normal eating.

What's more, the stress of yo-yo dieting is a threat to both life and health. Among women, yo-yo dieting has been shown to be *harmful to the immune system*. In a 2004 study of the relationship between weight and the activity of killer cells that destroy viruses and defend good cells, women with a history of repeated loss and regain of weight had one third less natural killer-cell capacity than women with a stable healthy weight. As for men, the well-known 1988 study tracking more than 11,000 Harvard alumni found markedly higher death rates from cardiovascular disease among men whose weight had gone up and down cyclically during adulthood.

But the reason is psychological too. A diet is an exception—a deviation from the norm. You go on a diet for two weeks so you can fit into that dress for New Year's Eve, and by January 2, you're ready to go back to your normal way of eating. Guess what? Your normal way of eating will bring you right back to the weight you were at before you deviated from the norm.

Where Dieting Backfires

The bottom line is that dieting is a short-term fix with adverse long-term implications. Yes, people lose weight on diets. The reason is simple: One way or the other, diets force them to take in fewer calories, and where weight loss is concerned, calories count.

Think about it: Whatever the theme of the diet, it constitutes some form of calorie lowering—either by depriving the dieter of certain kinds of food, by limiting portion size, or by requiring the dieter to eat at certain times rather than in response to feelings of hunger. Moreover, once people are on a diet and are eating only particular foods, for example, or are cutting out carbohydrates, or are measuring every bite, or are eating stringently small snacks five times a day when an alarm bell sounds, they tend to lose interest in eating. And not eating is certainly one way to lose weight.

But once the diet is over, of course, it is back to the foods the dieter dreamed of when she was cutting out carbs, or weighing every meal on a scale, or eating at three-hour intervals whether she felt like it or not. And that's when the weight comes back on.

Eating Well to Stay Well

The other downside of dieting is that *many diets—and certainly the most popular ones—put healthful eating second to weight loss. In fact, just as the way we eat is killing us, the way we diet may be killing us as well.*

Is there anyone who hasn't heard of the Atkins Diet? It requires almost complete avoidance of carbohydrates. During the initial phase of the diet—or whenever the weight loss slows—dieters are allowed no fruit, no beans, and very little in the way of vegetables. Yet those are foods that provide the nutrients essential for fighting disease and staying healthy. And what replaces them? *The Atkins Diet is all about animal proteins and fats—without distinguishing between the good proteins and fats that are essential for life and the bad proteins and fats that shorten your expected life span.* Simply put: This is a diet that increases the risk of all major diseases.

Its seemingly "healthier" version, the *South Beach Diet,* isn't much better. Based on glycemic index, it *rejects such fruits and vegetables as watermelon, beets, and carrots—with their health-promoting nutrients and the fiber* that make them so good not just for your health but for weight loss. And neither Atkins nor South Beach pays even lip service to the health benefits of soy or other plant protein. Instead, both diets advocate the liberal use of animal protein foods. (For a closer look at a day in the life of these diets, see the food demonstrations shown in the photo insert.)

No, diets don't do it. They fail both at achieving sustainable weight loss and at inculcating eating habits that help prevent disease and ensure good health. Dieting, in fact, has become the parallel lane on a two-lane highway that is taking Americans straight to overweight and ill health. It's time to get off that road. It's time to change direction.

Phyto Fighters Against Heart Disease Here is a rainbow of fruits and vegetables that help protect against heart disease:	
Phytonutrient	**Food Sources**
Carotenoids	Carrots, yams, cantaloupe, apricots, winter squash
Lycopene	Tomatoes, red grapefruit
Lutein	Spinach, kale, turnip greens
Capsaicin	Red chili peppers
Anthcyanins	Concord grapes, eggplant, red cabbage, radishes
Anthoxanthins	Cauliflower, potatoes
Betacyanin	Beets
Catechins	Green and black tea
Flavonols	Grape seeds
Flavonoids	Citrus fruit, berries, tomatoes, peppers
Lignans	Flaxseed, wheat, barley
Resveratrol	Grape skins
Ellagic acid	Strawberries, grapes, apples, cranberries, blackberries, walnuts
Glycerritinin	Licorice root

Dr. Shapiro's Picture Perfect Prescription Food Pyramid

What kind of eating will do that? Fortunately, as I've said before, *the same kind of eating that promotes weight loss most effectively is the kind of eating that promotes health and longevity.* And that is the kind of eating embodied in what I call the Picture Perfect Prescription Food Pyramid.

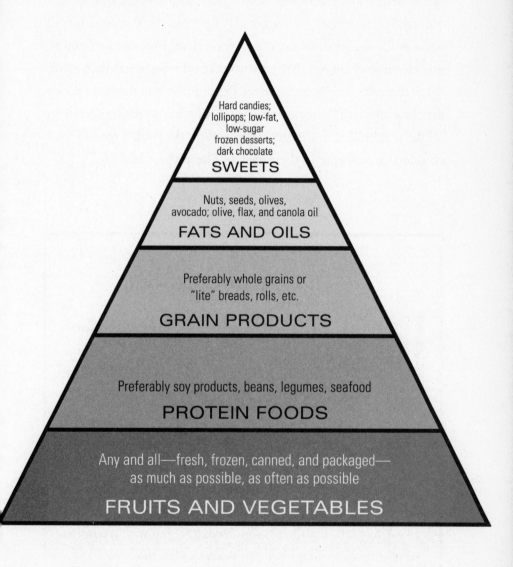

For over a quarter of a century, this pyramid has been the basis of my weight loss practice in New York. And for over a quarter of a century, it has worked for thousands of people. They come from all walks of life—celebrities and office workers, athletes and firefighters, housewives and lawyers. My patients take off weight and keep it off. Why? Because the Picture Perfect Prescription lets them eat foods they love and eat till they are satisfied. And it has worked to get them off the treadmill of unhealthy eating and on the golden road of food choices that will extend their lives and keep them healthy.

The Building of the Pyramid

The Picture Perfect Prescription Food Pyramid represents the results of all the latest research on the relationship between food and health and between eating and weight loss. From nutritional studies, we have complex new findings and conclusions that have been taken into account in creating this new Food Pyramid. Using this as your guide, you will be able to make instant food choices that are both nutritious and low calorie. The pyramid maps the proportionate representation of different kinds of foods in an overall eating plan. Eat the pyramid way, and you will maximize your good health and add ten years to your life.

Make fruits and vegetables the foundation of your eating.

Just as the pyramid is necessarily widest at the base, let fruits and vegetables be the foods you eat most—most often, most regularly, and most *of.* Your mother was right: These are the foods that are good for you. Whenever you get your fill of fruits and vegetables, you get their beneficial ingredients, which include:

- Fiber—Fiber works in many ways to clean and regulate the system. It's extremely important in *preventing many kinds of cancer, diabetes, heart disease, and obesity.* In overweight patients, fiber provides a feeling of being "full" that's the key to satisfying appetite.

The Top Seven High-Fiber Hits

Figs
Raspberries
Blackberries
Winter squash
Pumpkin
Avocado
Watermelon

- Vitamins—We hear so much about vitamins we forget why we need them. They act as powerful *prevention against disease and the aging process,* and of course, they are necessary for good metabolism and healthy living in general. The way we eat today—the way the Joneses eat—typically doesn't allow our bodies to keep up with our vitamin needs. We need to change the way we eat to take advantage of the vitamin power in fruits and vegetables.

- Minerals—Minerals are chemical elements required by living organisms. Take chromium, for example. We know that it's required for proper metabolism of sugar, and we know that inadequate chromium can affect the way insulin regulates sugar balance. Scientists are still exploring why this is true, but they know for sure that these elements are *essential for life. Vegetables and fruits are packed with minerals.*

- Phytonutrients—The rich colors of vegetables and fruits hold a deep and powerful mystery: the healing properties of their phytonutrients (sometimes called phytochemicals). Carotenoids, phenols, indoles, and isoflavones, to name just a few, help neutralize free radical damage and slow the aging process. Phytonutrients both *fight disease and promote health.* Clinical trials are finding that they *enhance the immune system, help prevent cancer, slow brain aging, and improve vision.* The benefits of these phytonutrients are as varied and as rich as the diversity of vegetables and fruits themselves.

The bottom line? Fruits and vegetables—fresh, frozen, canned, stir-fried, pickled, in soups, or any way you eat them—should be your base food. They're the bedrock on which you build your way of eating for health, slimness, and longevity.

Ah, Nuts!

Want to lose weight? Then forgive us if we say: Nuts to you! A recent weight reduction trial performed on sixty-five overweight or obese adults ranging in age from twenty-nine to seventy-nine gave all participants the same supervised meal plan, but in randomly chosen participants replaced complex carbohydrate foods with an equal-calorie amount of almonds. The result? The group on almonds lost more pounds around the waist (14 percent vs. 9 percent), fat mass (30 percent vs. 20 percent), total body water (8 percent vs. 1 percent), and systolic blood pressure (11 percent vs. 0).

Assume the same benefits for all other kinds of nuts.

Next, go for protein.

As I've already made clear, it's not animal protein you need. As often as possible, get your protein in beans and other legumes, fish and seafood,* and soy products rather than in meats, poultry, and dairy. Soy products can be particularly important. If any food deserves the label of "magic bullet" in terms of its power to fight disease and assist weight loss, that food is soy. Compounds in

---

* The government has warned about the mercury content and possible carcinogens in swordfish, shark, king mackerel, tilefish, and farm-raised salmon. Research on this issue is ongoing, so readers should "stay tuned" to the headlines. Wild salmon, sardines, herring, cod, sole, and other ocean fish are your best bets. In particular, salmon, sardines, and herring are rich in omega-3 fatty acids, which are good for the immune system, the neurological system, and the heart—and are thus much better for you than the saturated fats in meat, poultry, and dairy.

soybeans have been shown to protect bone strength, help prevent diabetes and kidney disease, stave off certain kinds of cancer, and actively promote weight loss. With food manufacturers catching on to the growing popularity of soy, soy-based food products are proliferating—and getting better-tasting—so you can now add soy dishes to breakfast, lunch, snacks, or dinner and enjoy both the taste and the extraordinary health benefits of this bean.

Soy vs. Cancer

In a study that included people from fifty-nine countries, researchers showed that the incidence of fatal prostate cancer was inversely related to the intake of soy products. In fact, soy was four times more likely to prevent prostate cancer than any other ingredient in the diet.

In Asian countries, where soy has long been a culinary staple, the incidence of breast and prostate cancer is far below that of Western countries. Recent studies in the United States, Japan, and China confirm that even one serving of soy per day can halve the risk of colon, rectal, lung, and breast cancer.

It has also been found that replacing dairy products with soy products can lower the risk of ovarian cancer. The substance in dairy products that increases the risk of ovarian cancer is galactose, a breakdown product of milk sugar, or lactose. Drinking soy milk instead of cow's milk and eating soy products in place of yogurt and other dairy products can therefore lower galactose intake and decrease your risk of ovarian cancer.

Recent studies have also shown that two substances that occur together in many dairy products—estrogen and IGF-1, an insulin-like growth factor—spur the growth of cancer cells, particularly breast and prostate cancer. Researchers found, for example, that men with higher levels of IGF-1 were more likely to develop prostate cancers than men with low levels of IGF-1. Again, substituting soy products for dairy products can lower this likelihood.

Next up the pyramid are grain products.

Select whole-grain or "light" versions if possible. Why? "Refining" these products quite simply takes the nutrients out of them. You lose the fiber, vitamins, minerals, and other phytochemicals that seem to work together to help reduce risk of heart disease, cancer, and diabetes. So look for the words "whole grain" or "100 percent whole wheat," for example, on the package of breads and cereals. Try some new kinds of grains to get the health benefits along with the richer taste of the real thing. Or go for the light breads; they are lower in calories than real bread, and a good source of fiber.

Fats and oils

Choose nuts, seeds, olives, avocado, and either olive or flax or canola oil wherever possible.

Good Fats

While saturated fat from animal foods and trans fat from hydrogenated oils can increase the risk of heart attack, stroke, and some forms of cancer, other fats are essential for health. They boost the immune and neurological systems, decrease the risk of heart disease and high blood pressure, help control diabetes, and can reduce inflammation in the body—including arthritis.

Here are good sources of healthy fats.

Monounsaturated Fats	Omega-3 Fats
Olive oil	Flax
Peanut oil	Fatty fish
Canola oil	Walnuts
	Soy

For sweet treats

Go for hard candies, lollipops, low-fat/low-sugar frozen desserts like Fudgsicles and Popsicles, and dark chocolate—a delicious and effective way to fight heart disease, although fairly high in calories.

See? It's really not hard to make the pyramid your main way of eating. On the contrary, it's as easy as living well and feeling good. Make it your guide, and you will live longer and be thin and healthy for life.

And if you want to know why I call it the Picture Perfect Prescription Pyramid, it's because it's best demonstrated in pictures. Read on.

Better Living Through Better Eating

The next eleven days will teach you how to eat the pyramid way. Simply put, you will change your relationship with food.

You will learn that there is an almost endless bounty of diverse, delicious, absolutely delectable food on our planet, so that you can always—always—make the healthful, low-calorie choice without ever sacrificing taste.

You will learn that food is not the enemy, that choice is not deprivation, and that deprivation is unnecessary. If you've ever been on a diet before and have sworn to yourself that you'll never again eat a hot fudge sundae / Southern fried chicken / Swiss fondue / chocolate cake / name your own food fantasy, you know how unrealistic such a vow is. And how foolish. Hot fudge sundaes are one of the joys of life, and it would be criminal to take an oath never to have one again. You *will* have one again, but when you do, it will be with awareness that this is a very high-calorie food, and that an occasional splurge does not equal a bad or unhealthy way of eating.

To gain this kind of awareness, you will expose yourself to new foods—especially in the first four days. You will also learn over the next eleven days that following the Picture Perfect Prescription Food Pyramid gives you a way of eating that is compatible with your way of life—whatever it is. You don't have to "give up" a business dinner, a restaurant, a New Year's Eve party, or a Fourth of July picnic. You won't feel like an outsider because of what you order in the company cafeteria or because of what's available in your pantry. You're not, after all, "on a diet." As I've emphasized, you're entering into a new relationship with food, and when that happens, you'll start a new way of eating. Whatever your lifestyle, whatever your tastes, whatever your needs, they fit into this new way of eating, and the new way of eating accommodates them.

Guidelines to
The Eleven-Day Program

Here's an eating plan for the next eleven days that will let you lose up to seven pounds, eat healthfully, and change your relationship with food. For the plan as a whole, keep the following guidelines in mind.

All the meals here are interchangeable, with the exception of the ones in the Three-Day Healthy Low-Carb Blitz. If there's a particular food you don't like, replace it with any food from the same rung of the pyramid—lentil soup for black bean soup, for example, or watermelon for berries.

Remember: No food is forbidden. *Our pyramid does not recommend meat, poultry, or dairy foods because we prefer healthier choices. But including these foods in your diet on occasion and in limited amounts is certainly acceptable.*

Also, the meals don't have to be homemade; eat them in a restaurant or do take-out if you prefer. And if you do cook at home, keep in mind that commercially prepared, packaged, or canned foods are just fine.

You'll note that you don't see beverages or condiments and

sauces in the program. Among beverages, you can stick to your favorites as long as they're coffee, tea, diet beverages, or sugar-free cocoa. For the milk you are using with cereal, coffee, and tea, the order of preference would be soy milk first, then skim milk, then one-percent milk.

The Pluses of Coffee and Green Tea

Not only does caffeine improve mental and physical performance, it also has some appetite-suppressing and calorie-burning properties. Bottom line? If there's no medical reason for eliminating caffeine from your diet, coffee is a good weight-loss tool.

As for green tea, it has a definite effect on calorie burning and is a boon to the immune system as well. Therefore, it is to be recommended as a weight-loss remedy. In fact, it's downright good for you. Here's a tip, though: It works best as a weight-loss remedy when taken with other caffeine, so pop a green-tea pill with a diet cola or a cup of tea or coffee, and you'll burn calories even more effectively.

For sauces, condiments, and marinades, check the following list to see the ones that add flavor, moisture, and versatility to any food at any meal.

- light salad dressings
- light mayonnaise

- mustards: Dijon, Pommery, and other kinds
- tomato purée, tomato paste, tomato sauce—including bottled pasta sauces
- clam juice, tomato juice, V8 vegetable juice, lemon or lime juice
- vinegars: balsamic, cider, wine, tarragon, etc.
- horseradish: red, white
- sauces: salsa, cocktail, tamari, soy, A-1, Worcestershire, barbecue, ketchup, duck sauce, black bean, hoisin, oyster, chutney, relish
- onion: fresh, juice, flakes, powder
- garlic: fresh, juice, flakes, powder
- herbs: all, especially basil, oregano, tarragon, thyme, rosemary, marjoram, dill, chives, sage, bay leaves
- spices: all, especially cinnamon, cloves, ginger, cumin, nutmeg, coriander, curry, paprika, allspice
- extracts: vanilla, almond, peppermint, maple, coconut
- cocoa powder
- broth, soups as sauces, marinades, or cooking liquids.
- Other soups preferably those with vegetables and/or beans, peas, or lentils

Red Wine and Heart Health: A Votre Santé!

Good news out of England, where a team of London-based scientists has concluded why and how red wine reduces the risk of heart disease. It's the polyphenols that do it—antioxidants that protect cells from damage. In this case, they're blocking a peptide that would otherwise constrict blood vessels. But only red wine does it; whites and rosés, say the English scientists, have no effect. And while red grape juice does exhibit some of the peptide-blocking properties of red wine, it proves to be "markedly less potent," according to the study.

Doing It Your Way

As for when and how much you should eat, eat when you're hungry, and stop eating when you're satisfied. If three full meals and two snacks a day is not your style, follow your habit. If you're not a breakfast eater, don't eat breakfast. If you usually skip lunch, keep on skipping it. If possible, don't miss more than one meal a day, but don't upset your own eating style too drastically. If weight loss is not a goal, be liberal with the grain products and other starchy foods, but try to use whole grains wherever possible.

You'll find a number of suggested recipes here, so that if you love to cook you can expand your eating options even further. The recipes start on page 187.

By the way, although the point really is to learn the principles of healthful, low-calorie eating for life, if you follow the plan laid out here, *you can lose seven pounds in the eleven days.*

EAT

THE ELEVEN-DAY PROGRAM

DAYS 1–4: THE AWARENESS DAYS

I've deliberately structured these first four days to challenge you to eat in a way you never have eaten before. You'll be following a program focusing on soy, fish, whole grains, soups, fruits, and vegetables. You may have avoided some of these foods before because you thought you disliked them. *But in the next four days, I want you to try them. That's all I ask!*

If you've got the daring to do so, you will find surprise after surprise. You'll discover foods that taste great. You'll find it's easy to eat them. You'll have increased energy. You'll lose weight. And the reward for all your daring? Simply this: a longer life.

The idea is to extend the range of foods you *like*. For that reason, there are two options for most of the suggested meals. There are also a number of foods that require preparation.

Chances are, you won't like every new food or recipe you try, but you will like some. And maybe you will also be prompted to try more new foods as a result. As I tell my patients: There is such an extraordinary variety of foods in the world, it's a shame to limit yourself to meat and potatoes.

After these four days of expanding options, I will offer an example of what a healthy, slimming seven-day eating plan could look like—day by day, meal by meal—including a three-day healthy, low-carb blitz.

I am going to ask you to try two servings of soy each day throughout the eleven days. I ask this for two reasons. First, I want you to get an idea of the variety of soy products out there so you can find versions of this terribly important food that can become an inherent part of the way you eat. Second, if you eat *two servings of soy foods per day*—preferably replacing meat or dairy choices—you *will lower your cholesterol* by anywhere from 10 percent to 17 percent while you also get the other disease-fighting, health-promoting, weight-loss benefits of this food. For a vivid demonstration of the difference soy can make, see the "The Soy Difference" chart on page 164.

	Fat grams	Saturated fat grams	Cholesterol mg	Calories	Soy protein grams	Fiber grams
Cooked beefburger	26	10	130	380	0	0
Cooked turkey burger	14	4	116	230	0	0
Veggie burger	2	0	0	180	26	4
Smoked pork sausage	22	8	50	280	0	0
Veggie smoked sausage	6	$\frac{1}{2}$	0	120	12	2
Cooked chicken breast with wing	15	5	120	300	0	0
Veggie chicken patty	5	0	0	200	26	6

The Soy Difference
(Each of the servings below is the same size—142 grams.)

Oil Change

Change the kind of oil you use in your salad dressing and you can also lower your blood pressure and favorably affect many of the other conditions of metabolic syndrome. (See pages 142–143.) Using any of the oils on the Picture Perfect Prescription Food Pyramid—olive, canola, flax, etc.—and even just eating fatty fish or flaxseed products can bring down both systolic and diastolic pressure. In fact, if Americans changed the oil they used, we could dramatically reduce the number of people now classified as "hypertensive," by as much as 40 percent.

The oil change can also increase insulin sensitivity, decrease fasting glucose levels, lower triglycerides, and raise your "good" cholesterol. In short, this is a lube job that can keep you running smoothly, free of metabolic syndrome.

Day 1: Try something new.

Today I ask you to try a food you've never eaten before or one you wouldn't normally have. The day's suggested menu offers a number of possibilities.

How about soy in the form of sautéed veggie breakfast links or patties? These are particularly tasty—and a great way to introduce soy into your diet.

Do you like steak? If so, you'll love the portobello mushrooms in today's lunch sandwich. Portobellos have a meaty texture, and the more you cook them, the meatier tasting they get. They can be prepared any number of ways—marinated and grilled, oven roasted, sautéed, stir-fried. They work well as salad toppings or accompaniments, or can be served as the main dish. Like all mushrooms, they are low in fat and calories and high in disease-fighting properties, especially for cancer prevention.

Another possibility this morning is to try some of the low-cholesterol egg products—such as Egg Beaters or Scramblers. Or you can make your own healthier version of scrambled eggs using egg whites.

Today it's also important that you start the day with fruit.

Here's the Day 1 expand-your-options menu:

Breakfast:
(option 1)
Mixed berries
Spanish omelet (use Egg Beaters, Scramblers, or egg whites with peppers, onions, olives, and tomato sauce)
Light or whole-grain toast

(option 2)
Mixed berries
Veggie (soy-based) breakfast links
Light or whole-grain pancake
Sugar-free or light syrup

Lunch:
(option 1)
Black bean soup
Veggie burgers with onion, tomato, pickles, and ketchup
Light or whole-grain bun

Tossed green salad with light dressing

(option 2)
Lentil or mixed bean salad on greens with tomatoes
Portobello mushroom sandwich on light or whole-grain roll

Snack:
Raw vegetables with hummus and/or salsa

Dinner:
(option 1)
Chinese: Hot-and-sour soup
      Mixed seafood with Chinese vegetables and hoisin, black bean, or ginger sauce (or Buddha's delight or vegetable chow mein)

(option 2)
Japanese: Miso soup
      Edamame
      Sashimi or seafood teriyaki

Snack or dessert:
Fresh strawberries with Almond-Mocha Fruit Dip

Results of Day 1: *You've begun to change your way of eating.*

Day 2: Focus on fish.
    Yes, it's true: We have so polluted our oceans and streams and waterways that much fish life is now unsafe to eat. Mercury

content and the presence of carcinogens have made swordfish, shark, king mackerel, tilefish, and farm-raised salmon pretty much forbidden foods for most of the population. Yet as proteins go— and proteins are of course essential in any eating plan—fish represents a far healthier choice than meat, poultry, or dairy.

Today's suggested menu offers fish choices at breakfast and lunch. Choose one.

Of course, if you really don't like fish, choose something else from the same rung of the pyramid. No problem.

Meanwhile, here's the suggested menu:

Breakfast:
(option 1)
Sliced orange
Smoked salmon (and/or sable, sturgeon, whitefish, etc.) on light or whole-grain roll with light or nondairy cream cheese

(option 2)
Sliced orange
Cold cereal (Cheerios, shredded wheat, bran flakes, or other whole-grain cereal)
Milk
Blueberries, banana

Lunch:
(option 1)
Three-bean chili with onions, salsa, and guacamole
Lemon-Poppy Carrot Salad on greens (page 191)

(option 2)
Mussels in marinara sauce
Grilled vegetables
Cucumber salad

Snack:
Roasted soy nuts

Dinner:
(option 1)
Barbecue/grill: veggie bratwurst, kielbasa, or Italian sausages
Mixed peppers
Sautéed mushrooms
Corn on the cob

(option 2)
Grilled or barbecued chicken
Mixed peppers
Sautéed mushrooms
Corn on the cob

Snack or dessert:
Watermelon

Results of Day 2: *You've chosen healthier foods as your sources of protein.*

Day 3: Send for soup; hail to whole grains.
A double focus today: the importance of soup and the benefits

of whole-grain foods.

I have long made soups a keystone of the weight-loss treatment I prescribe for my patients. They are a particular favorite with the many groups of New York City firefighters I've worked with, men who have lost an average of thirty-two pounds over a period of ten weeks. Being a firefighter, as I'm sure you know, means spending long hours on call in the firehouse, where firemen take their turns as head chef for the entire squad. Now, in firehouses around New York City, "graduates" of my program have become inventive soup chefs who turn out what are, in effect, hearty one-pot meals for burly guys with varied tastes who need to be well fueled and ready at all times.

But soups aren't just a meal-unto-themselves convenience. Canned, dried, or homemade, they're a great way to get your vegetables—especially if you're someone who thinks you don't like vegetables. Moreover, soups are a multipurpose food; use them as a marinade or to create a sauce. Finally, soups can unleash your culinary creativity: Experiment with ingredients, and spice up the results with condiments and herbs. You're limited only by your imagination.

As for the *whole grains*, they're what to look for—*in place of refined products*—when choosing breads and cereals. When you eat foods made with refined grains, vital nutrients and fiber have been removed. (It's done primarily to give those packaged foods a longer shelf life.) But refined-grain foods translate into greater risk for obesity and diabetes. It's a bad bargain. So, today, breakfast on whole grains or the light breads—filled with fiber and low in calories—and make them part of your way of eating for life.

Breakfast:
(option 1)
Ginger-Fruit Yogurt (page 190)
Light or whole-grain waffle
Sugar-free or light syrup

(option 2)
Cinnamon baked apple
Light or whole-grain toast
Peanut butter

Lunch:
(option 1)
Split-pea soup
Mixed vegetable salad (any vegetables—including pickled and/or marinated)
Light dressing
Toasted sunflower seeds

(option 2)
Tomato soup
Shrimp Caesar salad

Snack:
Low-carb chips (CarbFit, Keto—a good source of soy protein)

Dinner:
(option 1)
Baked Eggplant Casserole with Veggie Ground Beef (page 187)

Italian green beans
Marinated artichoke hearts

(option 2)
Veggie meatballs in marinara, puttanesca, or tomato-basil sauce
Italian green beans
Marinated artichoke hearts

Snack or dessert:
Orange and Spice Pumpkin Pudding (page 191)

Results of Day 3: *You've filled up on phytonutrients; you're fighting the killer diseases.*

Day 4: Eat your vegetables.
Today you're going to eat a range of vegetables of different textures, colors, and tastes. And you're going to bolster their health-promoting qualities with some soy products. Every day, more tasty soy products are distributed through supermarkets and health-food stores. So here are today's suggested meals:

Breakfast:
(option 1)
Cantaloupe or honeydew melon
Veggie sausage patties on light or whole-grain English muffin

(option 2)
Orange
Whole-grain hot cereal (oatmeal, Wheatena, etc.) with

chopped nuts and sugar-free syrup

Lunch:
(option 1)
Vegetable soup
Curried "Egg" Salad (page 188) sandwich on light or whole-grain bread   with lettuce and peppers (or commercially prepared veggie "egg," "chicken," or "turkey" salad)
Sliced tomatoes and avocado

(option 2)
Grilled vegetable plate
Baked sweet potato
Sliced tomatoes and avocado

Snack:
Roasted peanuts

Dinner:
(option 1)
Grilled tuna with lemon and herbs or teriyaki sauce
Baked acorn squash
Sweet-and-Sour Red Cabbage (page 196)
Cucumber dill salad

(option 2)
Veggie Buffalo wings or veggie chicken nuggets
Sweet-and-Sour Red Cabbage
Cucumber dill salad

Snack or dessert:
Low-calorie Creamsicle or Fudgsicle

Results of Day 4: *You've pushed the envelope. You've begun to change your entire relationship with food.*

DAYS 5–11: THE ACTION DAYS

Here is a seven-day example of an ideal eating program. What follows is a Picture Perfection Prescription for lowering your risk of major diseases significantly and adding years to your life. It's ideal also for maximum weight loss with maximum safety and healthfulness. I call it the **New Picture-Perfect Eating Plan with a Three-Day Healthy Low-Carb Blitz.** It follows all the principles of the Picture-Perfect Prescription Food Pyramid and is thus an example of what a healthy week's eating might look like—with the added goal of weight loss tossed in.

Be assured that if you follow the plan to the letter, you will, with every bite of food, lower your risk of disease. You will also set yourself up for weight loss—through four days of healthy, lower-calorie eating followed by another three days of healthy, low-carb, lower-calorie eating.

Let me say just a word or two about calorie reduction. It is one of the main keys to weight loss, which is why it is the basis of my medical practice. If you take a look at the food demonstrations shown in the photo insert, you'll get an instant picture of how daily food choices help you slash calories while you eat to your heart's content.

And now scientists have learned that you get more benefit from calorie reduction than mere weight loss. Animal research on calorie reduction—going on today in labs around the world—is confirming that restricting or reducing calorie intake can extend life expectancy and delay and/or mitigate the effects of aging and of age-related diseases. Part of the reason, of course, is that reducing body weight reduces the risk of obesity-related ailments. But researchers also conclude that reducing caloric intake may lower the production of free radicals that harm cells and may diminish a process called glycation, which alters protein structure and decreases biological activity, leading to a number of debilitating diseases.

All the results are not in yet—and there's more work to be done. But the results, so far, are conclusive, and they confirm the importance of *healthy calorie reduction as a way to lose weight, extend life, and improve its quality*.

The key word is *healthy* calorie reduction. As we have seen, *most diets don't fit the bill*. While many of the most popular diets are in fact "stealth" calorie-reduction plans, many of the foods these diets restrict contain important nutrients. And why sacrifice health to lose weight when you can lose weight healthfully instead?

Good Carbs

What constitutes a "good" carbohydrate? Unrefined whole grains and beans and all fruits and vegetables are good carbohydrates. They are excellent sources of the nutrients that fight disease, and they are also sources of fiber, which not only fights disease but also helps in weight loss by inducing a sense of satiety. Eating too many foods that are high in refined carbohydrates—white rice, refined cereals, cake, etc.—can raise blood sugar fast and generates too much insulin. It also makes you crave more carb-based foods.

That's why, over the next seven days, you will eat foods that are generally low in calories but high in nutritional value. Even if you choose to follow the Three-Day Healthy Low-Carb Blitz, you'll still maintain a high level of nutrition (in contrast to other low-carb programs). The reason the Blitz lasts for only three days is that following a low-carb diet for much longer can be restrictive. *The Blitz ensures that your short-term, low-carb program doesn't leave you deprived of nutritional necessities.*

The Blitz I've designed can safely and effectively be used as a quick weight-loss program for a particular event or special purpose—such as your high school reunion or your daughter's wedding. In fact, the entire seven-day program will serve as a weight-loss plan if you are now overweight. But once you are on the seven-day plan, and selecting your food according to the guidelines of the Picture Perfect Prescription Food Pyramid, you won't need another Blitz again. The results you get are just the beginning of a plan that will keep you slim and healthy for life.

Day 5: Strive for the ideal.

Breakfast:
Fresh fruit cup
Light pancake with light maple syrup
Sautéed veggie sausage patties

Lunch:
White bean soup
Grilled portobello mushroom sandwich on a whole-grain roll with lettuce, sliced tomato, and onion
Coleslaw

Snack:
Pistachio nuts

Dinner:
Shrimp cocktail
Pasta primavera
Broccoli rabe with garlic and oil

Snack or dessert:
Poached Pears with Sherry (page 194)

Results of Day 5: *You have just enjoyed a day of satisfying food with minimum intake of calories.*

Day 6: *Lower your risk of disease.*

Breakfast:
Banana and dried blueberries
Oatmeal with cinnamon and sugar-free syrup
Milk

Lunch:
Tomato-vegetable soup
Turkey sandwich on light bread with lettuce and mustard

Snack:
Roasted soy nuts

Dinner:
Peppered Sea Bass (page 193)
Grilled tomatoes
Green peas
Pickled beets and onions

Snack or dessert:
Individual No-Bake Cheesecakes (page 190)

Results of Day 6: *You are getting health benefits and minimum calories.*

Day 7: Lower your calorie intake.

Breakfast:
Raspberries
Light toast and peanut butter

Lunch:
Curried Pumpkin Soup (page 189)
Spinach salad with tuna, chickpeas, peppers, and onions with light French dressing

Snack:
Tootsie Pop Lollipop

Dinner:
Vegetarian Sloppy Joe on a light bun (page 196)
Grilled mushrooms and asparagus

Snack or dessert:
Mango

Results of Day 7: *Without repeating a single food choice, your low-calorie habit continues.*

Day 8: Eat the pyramid way.

Breakfast:
Grapefruit
Lox, eggs, and onions (Scramblers, Egg Beaters, or egg whites)
Light toast

Lunch:
Lentil soup
Grilled vegetable plate with baked sweet potato

Snack:
Edamame

Dinner:
Baked cod with tomatoes and onions
Green beans and baby carrots
Cucumber salad

Snack or dessert:
Chocolate-dipped fruit

Results of Day 8: *You are experiencing the wonderful variety of foods you can enjoy, using the pyramid as a guide.*

Day 9: Three-Day Healthy Low-Carb Blitz 1.

During the next three days, the following low-calorie menus also emphasize low-carb foods. While you're on the Low-Carb Blitz—on Days 9, 10, and 11—you will have a varied diet that emphasizes healthful, low-carb foods. If you choose not to go on the Low-Carb Blitz, choose any meals from Days 1 through 8.

Breakfast:
Omelet (Scramblers, Egg Beaters, or egg whites) with spinach, mushrooms, and veggie ham or bacon
1 slice low-carb toast

Lunch:
Vegetable-lentil soup
Tuna salad on mixed greens, with vinaigrette dressing

Snack:
Roasted almonds

Dinner:
Vegetable antipasto with roasted peppers, marinated artichoke hearts, and olives
Veggie meatballs and low-carb pasta with pesto
Sautéed zucchini

Snack/dessert:
Peanut Butter Delight (page 192)

Results of Day 9: *You have completed your first day of the Low-Carb Blitz.*

Do You Love Chocolate?

That's not all bad, as chocolate is good for your heart. The cocoa flavonols in chocolate help keep the blood vessels open and running smoothly and appear to prevent blood clotting. The result is to prevent high blood pressure and the clogged arteries that can cause heart attacks. As with all phytonutrients, the richer the color of the source food, the more nutrients are present, so in this case, the darker the chocolate, the more the flavonols—and the more there is to love. Of course, chocolate does have a pretty high calorie count. . .

Day 10: Three-Day Healthy Low-Carb Blitz 2.

Breakfast:
Low-carb cereal, hot or cold, with chopped walnuts and sugar-free syrup or low-calorie sweetener and milk

Lunch:
Grilled mushrooms
Veggie burgers and tomato
Garden salad with Sesame-Flax Dressing (page 195) and toasted pumpkin seeds

Snack:
Low-carb chips

Dinner:
Chinese vegetable soup
Stir-fried shrimp and broccoli with cashew nuts, soy sauce, and
Chinese mustard

Snack or dessert:
Low-calorie Popsicle

Results of Day 10: *The second day of the Low-Carb Blitz is over, but you don't have feelings of hunger.*

Day 11: Three-Day Healthy Low-Carb Blitz 3.

Breakfast:
Sautéed veggie sausage patties on low-carb toast or roll
Sliced tomato

Lunch:
Black bean soup
Grilled salmon
Roasted cauliflower and asparagus

Snack:
Celery, olives, and hearts of palm

Dinner:
Picture Perfect Chili (page 194)
Herbed green beans
Tossed salad with Dijon vinaigrette

Snack or dessert:

Low-carb carrot cake or chocolate cake (commercially prepared or from Mini-Carb cake mix)

Results of Day 11: *You've changed your relationship with food— and you're adding healthy years to your life.*

The Next Time You Do the Three-Day Healthy Low-Carb Blitz . . .

Choose from among these foods. Except where noted, eat as much or as little as you like.

Protein foods

Beans, lentils

Egg Beaters, Scramblers, egg whites

Fish and shellfish—fresh, canned, smoked, etc.

Nuts and nut butters

Seeds

Tahini

Tofu, edamame, roasted soy nuts

Veggie burgers (such as Boca Burgers, Recipe Basics, Morningstar Farms Grillers, or Veggie Recipe Crumbles) sausages, deli slices, etc.

Vegetables
Artichoke and artichoke hearts
Asparagus
Bamboo shoots
Broccoli and broccoli rabe
Brussels sprouts
Cabbage, green or red
Cauliflower
Celery
Cucumber
Eggplant
Green beans
Green pepper
Jicama
Kale
Leeks
Lettuce
Mushrooms
Pickles
Radicchio
Radish
Scallions
Spinach
Sprouts
Summer squash
Tomato
Water chestnuts
Zucchini

Fats, oils, dressings, and condiments

Vegetable, olive, nut, or seed oils

Olives and avocados

Sauces and dressings made from ingredients on this list, sych as guacamole, pesto, hummus, bean dips, etc.

Low-carb dressings and sauces

Herbs and spices, salt, soy sauce, vinegar, mustard

Beverages

Coffee, tea, all diet beverages, including diet cocoa mixes, diet sodas, diet lemonade, etc.

Also . . .

Low-carb breads, cereals, crackers, and snacks in moderation

Low-carb high-protein bars, chocolate bars, cakes, or cookies: maximum one serving per day

Low-cal sweeteners

Sugar-free chewing gum

Sugar-free Popsicles and Fudgsicles

Picture Perfect Recipes

Almond-Mocha Fruit Dip

1-oz. package instant sugar-free chocolate pudding
1 cup cold coffee (or $\frac{1}{2}$ cup coffee and $\frac{1}{2}$ cup water)
1 tsp. almond extract

Place all ingredients in a mixing bowl. Beat with an electric mixer at low speed for 1 minute. Serve with whole berries or any sliced fruit. Makes ten 2-Tbsp. servings; 12 calories per serving.

Baked Eggplant Casserole with Veggie Ground Beef

1 large eggplant ($1\frac{1}{2}$–2 pounds)
1 cup coarsely chopped onion
2–3 cloves garlic, chopped
1 Tbsp. olive or canola oil
1 tsp. salt
1 12-oz. package veggie ground beef (Boca Burger, Recipe Basics, or Morningstar Farms Grillers, Veggie Recipe Crumbles)
2 cups tomato-based pasta sauce
$\frac{1}{4}$ cup light creamy salad dressing (light creamy Italian, light Caesar, light ranch, etc.)
$\frac{1}{4}$ cup sliced olives
1–2 Tbsp. mixed herbs

Preheat oven to 375°F. Slice eggplant into approximately $\frac{1}{4}$ inch slices and arrange in a single layer on greased cookie sheets or foil pans. Combine onion, garlic, oil, and salt in a mixing bowl, and spread mixture evenly over eggplant slices. Bake for about 30 minutes, or until eggplant is fork-tender. Remove from oven and lower temperature to 350°F. In a mixing bowl, combine veggie ground beef, tomato sauce, light dressing, olives, and herbs until well mixed. Alternate layers of sauce mixture and eggplant in a large casserole or baking dish, beginning and ending with sauce. Bake for 20 minutes.

Makes six to eight servings; approximately 145 calories per serving.

Curried "Egg" Salad

1 14-oz. package extra-firm tofu, drained and chopped
$\frac{3}{4}$ cup chopped celery
$\frac{1}{4}$ cup chopped onion
$\frac{1}{4}$ cup chopped dill or parsley
$\frac{1}{3}$ cup light mayonnaise
1 Tbsp. mustard
2–3 tsp. curry powder (or to taste)
1 $\frac{1}{2}$ tsp. salt
Pepper to taste

Stir all ingredients together in a large mixing bowl until well blended. Refrigerate at least 30 minutes before serving.

Makes six half-cup servings; 110 calories per serving.

Curried Pumpkin Soup

$\frac{1}{2}$ cup chopped onion

$\frac{1}{2}$ cup chopped red or yellow bell peppers

$\frac{1}{2}$ cup chopped celery (including leaves)

1 Tbsp. olive or canola oil

$4\frac{1}{2}$ tsp. curry powder (or to taste)

1 15-oz. can pumpkin

1 cup soy milk

1 cup water

1 Tbsp. lemon juice

1 Tbsp. Splenda sweetener

$1\frac{1}{2}$ tsp. salt

2 Tbsp. chopped cilantro

Combine chopped onion, peppers, celery, and olive or canola oil in a medium saucepan. Sauté over medium heat about 5 minutes, or until vegetables are slightly tender. Stir in curry powder and cook another minute. Add pumpkin, soy milk, water, lemon juice, Splenda, and salt. Stir until well blended; cover pot and simmer over low heat for about 15 minutes. Pour into bowls; sprinkle with chopped cilantro and serve.

Makes about 5 cups; 85 calories per cup.

Note: Fresh or frozen pumpkin or winter squash may be substituted for canned pumpkin.

Ginger-Fruit Yogurt

1 6-oz. container plain soy yogurt
$\frac{1}{2}$ cup diced fruit—apples, bananas, peaches, strawberries, etc.
1 Tbsp. Splenda sweetener
$\frac{1}{2}$ tsp. vanilla extract
$\frac{1}{2}$ tsp. ground ginger

Stir all ingredients together in a mixing bowl until well blended. Refrigerate at least 30 minutes before serving.

Makes one serving; 180 calories per serving.

Individual No-Bake Cheesecakes

4 ozs. nondairy cream cheese (e.g., Tofutti brand)
1 16-oz. package soft silken tofu
$\frac{1}{3}$ cup lemon juice
1 tsp. vanilla extract
$\frac{1}{2}$ tsp. grated lemon peel
$\frac{1}{4}$ tsp. salt
1 1-oz. package instant sugar-free vanilla pudding
Cinnamon
Strawberry slices for garnish, if desired

Process cream cheese, tofu, lemon juice, vanilla, lemon peel, and salt in an electric blender until smooth. Add pudding mix and blend until well incorporated. Spoon mixture into four foil muffin cups, custard cups, or dessert dishes, dividing evenly. Refrigerate at least 1 hour before serving. Sprinkle cinnamon on top, and garnish with strawberry slices, if desired.

Makes four half-cup servings; 185 calories per serving.

Lemon-Poppy Carrot Salad

2 cups shredded carrots
$\frac{1}{4}$ cup lemon juice
2 Tbsp. light mayonnaise
2 Tbsp. light French dressing
4 tsp. Splenda sweetener
2 tsp. poppy seeds
$\frac{1}{2}$ tsp. grated lemon peel
$\frac{1}{2}$ tsp. salt

Stir all ingredients together in a mixing bowl until well blended. Refrigerate at least 1 hour before serving.

Makes five half-cup servings; 60 calories per serving.

Orange-and-Spice Pumpkin Pudding

1 15-oz. can pumpkin
1 1-oz. package instant sugar-free vanilla pudding
$\frac{3}{4}$ cup water
1 Tbsp. lemon juice
1 Tbsp. brandy or rum (optional)
1 tsp. cinnamon

½ tsp. pumpkin pie spice
½ tsp. grated orange peel
¼ tsp. salt
Mint leaves and dollop of whipped topping for garnish, if desired

Combine all ingredients (except garnish) in a mixing bowl and beat with an electric mixer at low speed for about 1 minute. Spoon into dessert dishes and refrigerate at least 1 hour before serving. Garnish with mint leaves and whipped topping, if desired.

Makes four half-cup servings; approximately 65 calories per serving.

Peanut Butter Delight

4 Tbsp. peanut butter—chunky or creamy
1¾ cups water, divided
¼ tsp. salt
1 1-oz. package instant sugar-free butterscotch pudding (chocolate or vanilla pudding may be substituted)
Chopped peanuts for garnish, if desired

Place peanut butter * and ¾ cup water in an electric blender and process until smooth. Add remaining 1 cup of water, salt, and pudding mix and blend at low speed for about 1 minute. Spoon into dessert dishes and refrigerate at least 30 minutes before serving. Garnish with chopped peanuts, if desired.

Makes four half-cup servings; 115 calories per serving.

*We recommend natural peanut butter made only from peanuts and salt; it offers better peanut flavor and nutrition. Commercial brands, however, are fine if you can't get the natural version or if you prefer the taste (even though they contain trans fat). We do not recommend the reduced-fat versions; most of them contain significant amounts of refined carbohydrates.

Peppered Sea Bass

1 lb. Chilean sea bass, or other firm-fleshed fish fillet, cut into 4 pieces
2–3 Tbsp. mustard
Salt to taste
2–3 Tbsp. crushed peppercorns
1 Tbsp. olive or canola oil
Lemon wedges

Coat all sides of fish with mustard. Sprinkle with salt and peppercorns, patting evenly onto surface of fish. Heat oil in a large skillet over medium-high heat. Add fish and cook about 5 minutes on each side, or until fish is golden brown. (If fish fillets are very thick, transfer to a hot oven [375°F–425°F]) and cook for an additional 5 or 10 minutes, or until fish flakes with a fork. Serve with lemon wedges.

Makes four servings; approximately 170 calories per serving.

Picture Perfect Chili

1 cup coarsely chopped bell peppers—any color

1 cup chopped onion

3–4 cloves chopped or minced garlic

1 Tbsp. olive or canola oil

1 12-oz. package veggie ground beef (Morningstar Farms Grillers)

1 15-oz. can black or red beans, drained

1 15-oz. can chili beans in sauce

1 15-oz. jar tomato-based pasta sauce (Aunt Millie's, Prego, etc.)

1 14-oz. can diced tomatoes

1 4-oz. or 5-oz. can chopped green chilies

1 Tbsp. chili powder

1 Tbsp. dried oregano leaves

$\frac{1}{2}$ tsp. ground cumin

Sauté peppers, onions, and garlic in oil in a large skillet or saucepan over medium-high heat for 2 minutes. Stir in veggie ground beef and cook for another 2 minutes. Add all remaining ingredients and stir well. Bring to a boil; reduce heat to medium-low; cover pan and simmer for 20 minutes, stirring occasionally.

Makes about ten 1-cup servings; approximately 150 calories per serving.

Poached Pears with Sherry

5–6 large, ripe pears
2 cups water
1 cup Splenda sweetener
½ cup medium-dry sherry
2 Tbsp. lemon juice
2–3 cinnamon sticks

Wash, halve, and core pears; peel, if desired. Place all of the ingredients in a medium saucepan. Bring to a boil over high heat; cover pot, turn heat to low, and simmer for about 20 minutes, or until pears are fork-tender. Serve hot or cold.

Approximately 100 calories per serving (2 pear halves and ¼ cup liquid).

Note: Apples (5–6), peaches (7–8), or plums (8–10) may be used instead of pears.

Sesame-Flax Dressing

¼ cup toasted sesame oil
¼ cup flax oil
¼ cup vinegar
¼ cup mustard
¼ cup water
1 Tbsp. Splenda sweetener
½ tsp. salt
Pepper to taste

Stir all ingredients together in a mixing bowl until blended. Store in the refrigerator. If mixture separates, shake before serving.

Makes ten 2-Tbsp. servings; 90 calories per serving.

Sesame-Flax Dressing may also be used as a marinade.

Sweet-and-Sour Red Cabbage

1 medium-large head red cabbage (about 2–3 pounds), shredded
2 cups water
$\frac{3}{8}$ cup Splenda sweetener
3 Tbsp. vinegar—any kind
3 Tbsp. lemon juice
1 Tbsp. olive or canola oil
$\frac{1}{2}$ tsp. salt

Combine all ingredients in a large saucepan. Bring to a boil over high heat; reduce heat to medium, cover pot, and continue cooking for about 20 minutes, or until cabbage is tender and most of the liquid is evaporated.

Makes about eight cups; approximately 40 calories per cup.

Vegetarian Sloppy Joes

1 cup chopped onion

1 Tbsp. olive or canola oil

1 12-oz. package veggie ground beef (Morningstar Farm Grillers)

1 cup tomato-based pasta sauce (Aunt Millie's, Prego, etc.)

$\frac{1}{2}$ cup barbecue sauce

1 Tbsp. vinegar

Sauté onion in oil in a large skillet over medium heat for about 5 minutes, or until translucent. Stir in veggie ground beef, tomato sauce, barbecue sauce, and vinegar. Cook over medium heat for another 5 minutes, or until mixture is bubbly.

Makes about six 1-cup servings; 110 calories per serving, not including bun.

Making the Connection

Awareness			
DAY 1	**DAY 2**	**DAY 3**	**DAY 4**
How's your social health?	Get ready to get connected.	Assess your connectedness capability.	Change the tape in your head.

Action						
DAY 5	**DAY 6**	**DAY 7**	**DAY 8**	**DAY 9**	**DAY 10**	**DAY 11**
Serve your community.	Campaign for a cause.	Make a spiritual connec-tion.	Connect with the natural world.	Be with friends; reach out to family.	Join something.	Do for others.

Chapter 5

MAKING THE CONNECTION

When I talk about connectedness, I mean reaching beyond yourself to engage with other people and with the world at large. On this topic, it seems that literature has as much to say on the subject as science.

It was in 1624 that poet John Donne gave English speakers the great phrases that describe the interconnectedness of all people. "No man is an island, entire of itself; Every man is a piece of the continent, a part of the main," Donne wrote. The poet offered both an explanation and a watchword for this interconnectedness: "Any man's death diminishes me," he asserted, "because I am involved in mankind; and therefore never send to know for whom the bell tolls; it tolls for thee."

About three centuries later, novelist E. M. Forster addressed the same theme. "Only connect!" Forster urged in his 1910 novel, *Howards End.* "Live in fragments no longer." In connecting, Forster claimed, people become "exalted." They fulfill and elevate their humanness by answering the need to engage with others.

But it's not just literary figures who have noted the human

need to be connected. Science confirms that every one of us has a need to engage with others. In fact, as I've pointed out, it's one of the key life-expansion factors contributing to energetic good health and longevity.

But what are the best ways to get connected and stay connected?

Getting Connected in Eleven Days

In the eleven-day program, the first four days are designed to help you become more aware of the ways in which you're already connected. It's important to acknowledge and respect the connections you already have. At the same time, in those days you may begin to realize that there are a number of things you can do to increase your sense of connectedness and overcome some of the barriers that may be keeping you from opportunities for contact or relationships.

In the *Awareness* part of the program, I provide easy evaluations to help you get a snapshot of how connected or isolated you feel. I also help you check out your own preferences—that is, *discover the ways that you would like to be more connected*. (Some of these are surprisingly easy.) By the third and fourth days, as you evaluate where you are and what you would like to do, you will begin to *formulate a plan of action*.

In the *Action* part of the eleven-day program (the fifth day through the eleventh), you will find suggestions to help you explore your connections with friends, community, family, and the world at large.

In designing this program, I have once again turned to my colleague psychotherapist Susan Amato. Her review of the research, combined with the individual and group work that she has done, have made it possible for people to experience some remarkable turnarounds on the eleven-day program.

Feeling connected is far more than a change in your outlook. It is a way to invest your life with renewed energy and protect your health. The impact on quality of life and longevity is nothing less than remarkable.

What Research Shows

Study after study confirms the need for connectedness.

First of all, there's ample proof that having social support—*being part of a larger network of friends and family—has a profound impact on how long and how well you can expect to live.* In a Swedish study of fifty-year-old men who had endured high levels of emotional stress, *researchers found that those who lacked social support had a significantly shortened life expectancy.* When they checked the statistics, doctors concluded that these socially isolated men were three times more likely to die within the next seven years than were those who had ample emotional support and good relationships.

Not surprisingly, the same applies to women. A study published in 2003 of more than 7,500 women aged sixty-five and older found that those with large social networks—someone to talk to about decisions, people to provide help with daily chores—could be expected to live at least one to two years longer than women who were more isolated. And that was true even when severe medical conditions were taken into account.

This was further supported by a study that tracked 7,000 Californians over the course of seventeen years. Doctors found that those without meaningful social connections were almost 300 percent more likely to die prematurely than those who felt more socially connected.

Even when people have health problems, life improves—and so does life expectancy!—if there is significant social support. A study of nearly 1,400 people with heart disease found that those who were married or who had a significant other in their lives were far more likely to outlive heart-disease patients who had no one to confide in.

Studies also show that social contact is a strong vote for longer living. For instance, a Duke University study tracking 4,000 people over four years found that weekly churchgoers had a 28 percent lower mortality rate than those who did not join in the church community. At first, researchers thought it might be religious factors that made the big difference. But when they sorted through the evidence, they found that the leap in longevity was attributed not to religion per se but to the sense of connectedness offered by the church community. It turns out that, statistically, a person's chance of dying in the next year is cut in half when the individual joins a group or becomes a member of an organization.

The insurance companies have done thorough studies of those who live to age one hundred or over. Considering all factors, *actuaries report that social connectedness to family, friends, and social groups is a key "marker" of these long-lived centenarians.* Any insurance underwriter trying to assess a person's life expectancy and chances of successful aging pays a lot of attention to factors like a close-knit family or community, social contacts, and participation in group activities. These are key indicators of long life.

Toward a Longer, Happier Life

I've seen the phenomenon firsthand. As a doctor, I know that patients with strong personal relationships and social support are more likely to survive and bounce back more quickly from surgery, a heart attack, or catastrophic illness.

Heart attacks are more frequent among those forced into mandatory retirement, compared with people who keep working or immediately get involved with other pursuits. In fact, post-retirement heart attacks are so common that doctors consider their occurrence a medical syndrome. We know it isn't the *work* that retirees miss. They miss the *community* of work—the sense of shared purpose, and the feelings of support that are communicated among people who spend their days together. Take that away, as mandatory retirement does, and the result is, literally, a feeling of social deprivation. The body reacts dramatically.

I've also seen many examples of premature death among men who become particularly isolated. Social scientists tell us that divorced men die sooner than their ex-wives because they lack the network of close friends women tend to build.

In long marriage relationships, men often rely on the bond with their wives for connectedness, and vice versa. It is not uncommon for widows as well as widowers to die within a year of their spouses.

I find it interesting that so many scientists in the fields of medicine, sociology, and psychology agree that the *failure to connect shortens life and brings on the aging process*, yet none is able to explain why. We know that *isolation seems to depress the immune system*, making us more vulnerable to disease and even to accidents, but we don't fully understand the physiological mechanism behind that process. We know that depression often accompanies isolation, and it can trigger a loss of self-worth. People need a sense of purpose. (People who suffer isolation may actually stop eating and lose the will to live.) But the explanations for that are more intuitive than scientific.

Scientists continue to study the subject. No doubt, some day they will be able to trace the neurological, hormonal, and biological pathways that energize our minds and bodies, giving us the ability, desire, and will to live longer. In the meantime, all we know is that *it is a fact that reaching out to other people—staying in contact with a world outside ourselves—helps keep us young and adds years to our lives.*

Isolation, Not Aloneness

Before you start to think I'm saying that being alone is a bad thing, I'd like to emphasize the distinction between the kind of isolation that social scientists are talking about and feelings of independence, solitude, or aloneness that can be completely enjoyable. There is nothing unhealthy about being alone. In fact, reserving time for solitude—"enjoying your own company," as the expression goes—is just as necessary for human health as is connectedness. To be isolated, however, is to be set apart from others and to be cut off from any external influences.

You can be alone without feeling at all isolated. To take an extreme example, what about a lone monk living in a bare cell who has taken a vow of silence? Though living in solitude, he remains thoroughly connected to the world through study and thought, by corresponding with others, and of course through his deep faith and connection with God. It is equally possible for someone with a wide network of acquaintances, someone who is constantly busy, someone who is always surrounded by people, to be utterly unconnected to the world and to others. In the case of such a person, quantity of connections has perhaps obscured the lack of a quality relationship.

The Benefits of Being Connected

Just as it is essential to understand what isolation really is, it is equally important to understand what being connected is all about. To connect is, of course, to join, to link up with someone. Hidden inside the word is the notion of reciprocity—the idea that people at both ends of the connection are "exalted," as E. M. Forster said.

That's why being connected is so very important to keeping us young and helping us live longer.

In the most practical terms, of course, going out and participating with others is a way to meet people, develop supportive relationships, and make friends or create the foundation of an intimate relationship. It thus creates the opportunity for us to be comforted in tough times, helped during illness or crisis.

Being connected provides perspective; it takes us beyond the confining limits of isolation and lets us put ourselves, our stresses, and our successes in balance. That, in turn, provides us a framework for setting priorities that make sense in our lives.

But for many people, *it's just as beneficial to be connected to something as to someone.* In the way an avid chess player is connected to the game, a dedicated musician feels connected to music, or a lover of the outdoors finds connection through nature, there are many avocations as well as vocations that help people connect with something outside themselves. There is also the connectedness of sharing an interest with others, as when you join a cause in a common purpose, take part in religious worship, or hone your card-playing skills with a group of companions. You benefit doubly, both from getting connected and from bringing value to the connections you make.

In whatever way you "become connected," be sure to respect how important this is in your life. The time that you give to

socializing or pursuing things that interest you is the best insurance
you can have for a longer and healthier life. The results are
formidable in terms of enhancing and extending life.

Connected Kids

A study in the September 2004 issue of *Journal of Public
Health* found that high school students who feel more connected to their school get better grades than students who
don't share the feeling. The connected students also have
lower rates of absenteeism and drop out far less frequently.
Researchers found other attributes among students who
have a strong sense of affiliation with their schools—they
are far less likely to join gangs or use drugs or alcohol.

Ways to Connect

Since connectedness takes so many forms, you probably have
more opportunities than you realize. In the **Awareness** section of
the eleven-day program, you'll have a chance to weigh each of these
opportunities for yourself. Here are some things to consider:

- *Your relationships with spouse, partner, and friends.* The close
  connection between two people is a commitment that can
  take the form of marriage, long partnership, or close friend-
  ship. Whatever name you give it, this kind of relationship is

usually a boon to good health (yes, even with the inevitable ups and downs!). What matters is having someone to confide in. True, two people rarely share all of their worries, fears, hopes, dreams, complaints, and deepest thoughts. But if there's someone who won't judge you—someone you can trust—that's a very important part of feeling connected.

- *Your work.* People often feel connected to others through their work (though, as I've pointed out, some people don't realize its value until they retire!). The community of work might include colleagues at the office, in the field, or on the factory floor. Camaraderie is established when you join coworkers or colleagues in working toward a common goal. It gives you a sense of connectedness that goes beyond mere employment. After all, you spend about a third of your life with these people, and you're connected to each other by experiences, buzzwords, some similar interests, and loyalties.

- *Your affiliations.* People are united, and sometimes closely connected, by their affiliations with religious, political, or community organizations.

- *Your hobbies and avocations.* People form communities around shared interests, whether the local theater group, a jazz ensemble, the garden club, a quilting group, golf, or an Internet chat group about fifteenth-century Italian architecture.

- *Human aid and volunteer work.* People connect when they reach beyond themselves to do good works—when they volunteer to staff the sign-up table at the 5K run benefiting the local health center; when they deliver Meals on Wheels; when they grab a hammer and build houses with Habitat for Humanity; when they work at an animal shelter; when they go halfway around the world to help an aid organization try to save lives after a disaster; when they do volunteer work in hospitals. People feel connected when they campaign for a cause in which they believe.

• *Spiritual connectedness.* When you feel yourself united to a higher power or to a spiritual realm of life—even if you are all by yourself—you are connected.

The manner of connectedness doesn't matter. However you connect—however you engage with the world people live in—you link yourself to the lives of others. The effects are beneficial.

Psychologist Erich Fromm has noted: "The kind of relatedness to the world may be noble or trivial, but even being related to the basest kind of pattern is immensely preferable to being alone."

It is not just preferable to be connected; it is essential for extending your life span to its full potential, and for living as healthfully as possible right now.

That's why I ask you to take the next eleven days to examine your own level of connectedness and to take action to affirm, enhance, and expand this essential life extender.

Connecting Through Music

Does it seem eerie to see people walking along completely engrossed in the music on their CD or MP3 players, utterly isolated from one another? Many people enjoy feeling connected to music, and it's a powerful form of communication in itself. But soon there may be another way to connect not just with music itself but with other listeners who are nearby.

A device now under development at the Media Lab in Dublin, is aimed at letting all those solo listeners share the music. The aim of the prototype system, called tunA, is to create social connections among people who otherwise might not interact. If the prototype works, tunA users will be able to tune into the playlists of anyone within a radius of 1,600 square feet and listen in. An instant-messaging feature will even let them communicate with one another, although not by talking aloud, of course.

CONNECT

THE ELEVEN-DAY PROGRAM

DAYS 1–4: THE AWARENESS DAYS

Maybe you are always part of a crowd. Or perhaps you're a real loner. Maybe you're married, secure in a good, steady job, up to date on current affairs, outgoing and friendly, resident of a lively town or city. Or perhaps you work at home, in seclusion, in a remote rural area where you see your neighbors only rarely.

None of these characteristics really tells you whether or not you are connected to the world beyond yourself. So the first task of the eleven-day program is to ascertain whether and to what extent you may be isolated. But even if your self-evaluation during the first four days tells you that you have a healthy level of connectedness, I still suggest you look at the action steps in Days 5 through 11. There are some ideas there that you might want to use in the future even if at this moment you're right where you want to be.

Of course, if the awareness that you acquire in the first four days leads you to the conclusion that you really do need to be more connected and less isolated, then the seven days of action steps are more essential. You'll find out how you can begin to break out of your isolation and expand your connectedness.

Day 1: How's your social health?

Today you'll measure your own social connectedness. Here's a questionnaire that will let you know how strong your support system is, whether you feel part of a community, and how close your relationships are. For each question in the test, answer True or False.

True	False	
		1. I am invited out or have friends over at least every other week.
		2. My family and I are in touch regularly— certainly once a month.
		3. There is someone with whom I can share my troubles and triumphs.
		4. I regularly participate in my religious group or in a group with caring, supportive values.
		5. If I needed money on short notice, I definitely know at least one person I could call on for an emergency loan.
		6. There is no one in my life who really cares about my work and my achievements.
		7. I would have trouble finding someone to spend a day going shopping with me, much less to accompany me on a two-week vacation.
		8. If I needed to be met at the airport, I would call a cab; there's no one I know well enough to ask such a favor.
		9. Although I think I have a lot of love to give, there is no one in my life to whom I can express my love, caring, and concern.

For every True answer to questions 1 through 5, give yourself one point. For every False answer to questions 6 through 9, give yourself one point. Now add up your totals:

True (1–5): _____ False (6–9): _____ = Total: _____

Here's how your social health measures up:

If you scored . . .	you have . . .
8–9	A high level of connectedness—keep it up, make it even stronger to add years to your life.
6+	An adequate level of connectedness—but not enough to add appreciably to your life span.
5	An insufficient level of connectedness in your life—you would benefit greatly and add years to your life by reaching out beyond yourself.
4	A very low level of connectedness—you need to reach beyond yourself to end your isolation. (At this level, there's a very real risk that you'll shorten your life span if you continue with the same pattern.)

Results of Day 1: *You've identified your level of connectedness or isolation.*

Day 2: *Get ready to get connected.*

"I'm not a joiner."

"I like my solitude."

"I don't make friends easily."

"I haven't time to volunteer . . . to get involved . . . to participate. . . to help out . . ."

None of these statements is entirely honest. Yet words like these are often used as excuses to avoid taking risks, feeling embarrassed, or taking on new ventures. Unfortunately, such blanket statements need to be challenged—by you, if no one else. You're not helping yourself if you subscribe to belief statements that have little foundation in reality.

People who contend they are not "joiners," for the most part, have never made an attempt to join anything. People who claim they like their solitude often wish they could break out of it. People saying they don't make friends easily might not realize that there's often some level of difficulty in making friends. (But it's worth the effort!) And those who claim they haven't time to pursue anything other than their own purposes probably should make the time. (Remember, this isn't time-wasting—it's life-expanding.)

All the same, I'm not insisting you have to join anything, or give up your solitude, or introduce yourself to strangers, or volunteer. All these steps can help, but they aren't essential to being connected. Each person connects in his or her own individual way, in accord with his or her own style, and in a way that does not greatly upset his or her comfort level.

Two things are major determinants of how a person will connect: interest and time. *So, today, you are going to examine some categories of connectedness to see which might best fit you*—with your particular set of interests and inclinations. I would like you to look realistically at the amount of time you'll have to commit in order to begin connecting.

Below is a set of categories. To the extent that you get involved with these spheres of interest, you have the opportunity to feel more connected. Each kind of pursuit offers a great chance to move beyond the confines *of you* to link up with others.

As you look at the categories, assess your personal level of interest. Rate your interest on a scale of from 1 to 10.

In the Notes column, jot down the specific nature of your interest. For example, you might feel you are now ready to work for a cause, and the cause you would like to work for is environmental quality. Make a note of that.

Category	Level of Interest 1–10	Notes	Time Commitment
Spiritual/religious			
Volunteer work			
Friends			
Community			
Nature			
Cause			
Family			
Charity			
Hobby			

These categories are only a beginning. But be sure to *go through the exercise of filling out this form*. At first glance, you may be somewhat overconfident in judging which category interests you the most, and which the least. But I would wager that as you start filling out this form, you will surprise yourself with ideas that come to mind. You may be intrigued to find out how much you like the notion of getting involved and giving more time, particularly if you have a strong interest in one area. For many people, this evaluation is a big help in discovering how to reach out farther than ever before.

Now, without giving yourself any particular "assignment," think about how much time you can give to the effort to reach out. Be realistic; it is better to start small and work your way up than to think big and have to draw back. *Write your time commitment in the last column.*

Results of Day 2: *You have declared your strongest areas of interest and decided how much time you will commit. You are*

ready to reach out beyond yourself to connect to the wider world.

Day 3: Assess your connectedness capability.

Everybody is worthy of becoming connected. Everybody has something worthwhile to contribute. Whatever you bring, whether a strong pair of hands or special expertise, it is enough. Whatever your personality or passion, it's perfectly suited to engaging with the world. Today, you need to convince yourself of that.

To do so, *think about three things you succeeded in doing* even though you doubted your own capabilities at first. Maybe you went to a party that you were truly terrified of attending. Or perhaps you managed to ask your boss for a raise, even though you dreaded the encounter. Or you stood up in the public meeting and objected to a rezoning variance, risking the wrath of some neighbors.

Write down all three things.

Then analyze how you succeeded in overcoming your doubts, fears, and hesitations in order to do those things. If it was a party you dreaded, did you rehearse in your mind opening gambits for party conversation? If you finally had a long-deferred meeting with your boss to ask for a raise, did you write down your arguments and persuasions beforehand? If you stood up in a public meeting and challenged a zoning variance, did you research the zoning laws so you could quote them at the meeting?

Be as precise as possible about the steps you took to accomplish each seemingly difficult, scary, overwhelming thing. *Then write down those steps.*

Now remember that in each case you did the thing you didn't think you could do—and it was okay. Maybe you didn't enjoy the party, and maybe you didn't get the raise, and maybe you lost the zoning fight—or maybe not. But win or lose, you did the difficult thing and were not broken by it. In fact, if you look at what's on your list, I'll bet you are now glad that you expended your energy, whatever the outcome. Aren't you?

Having this assurance—which was proven by your own ability to take action—will be a great help as you take steps to become more connected.

Results of Day 3: *You have shown yourself that you can take action to improve your connectedness.*

Day 4: Change the tape in your head.

Do you know why people—maybe you included—may be reluctant to reach out and make connections? If you could see what was going on inside their heads, you'd find that 90 percent of the time, they simply feel afraid.

There are many things *we fear—embarrassment, looking foolish, being subjected to humiliation.* Whatever the source of our fears, *they can be formidable barriers.* Some people are afraid they'll be too embarrassed to approach a stranger at a party. Others fear they'll look foolish if they ask to volunteer at the local soup kitchen. Still others fear being humiliated by an indifferent response—being told, for instance, that they're not really needed on a certain team or committee. Often, the fear of rejection overrides every other impulse, even the best ones.

Of course, anyone who fears rejection is absolutely right. *Rejection is a possibility.* In fact, sometimes when you reach out, there's absolutely no doubt that you *will* be rejected. Count on it. But that's the way it is. *Rejection is a part of life.*

But isn't that good news, after all? If you're rejected, *it doesn't mean there's something wrong with you. It only means that you asked and were turned down. And everyone has that experience.*

Think of actors who must audition nearly every day of their lives. At ninety-nine out of one hundred auditions, they'll be told: "Thank you for coming in, but you're not what we're looking for." If at the first rejection, an actor says to himself: "That's it. I tried. It didn't work. I can stop now," he simply won't be around for that all-important one-hundredth audition when the director says, "Thank you. You're perfect. Sign here."

In my profession of medicine, one of the toughest problems to diagnose is appendicitis. The symptoms are almost never clear cut. When a doctor reviews symptoms, gathers evidence, and decides to operate, he or she is often right. That is, most of the time the lab tests lead a physician to make a diagnosis of appendicitis and to conclude that surgery is necessary. So the doctor makes the right decision. But in a certain percentage of cases, the doctor gets it wrong. Surgery is performed, and there is no sign of infection.

The question is, should a doctor avoid doing appendectomies just because he or she might make a mistake?

The slogan among doctors is that if it's positive every time you cut, you're doing something wrong. There must be negatives; they are simply part of the process. If a physician is prudently advising the safest course of action for his or her patients, then that physician will go ahead and perform surgery whenever all the symptoms point to appendicitis. Not to operate puts the patient's life at risk and is unacceptable. True, the physician will be wrong sometimes, and a healthy appendix will be removed. But that's an acceptable risk.

Being rejected or coming up negative—whether it's ninety-nine times out of one hundred if you're an actor, or one time out of twenty if you're a surgeon trying to save your patient—is an acceptable risk. What's your risk of being rejected in a particular situation? Whatever it is, it's acceptable, since a certain amount of rejection is just part of the process of living.

But what if you can't accept that fact? What if you feel as if rejection is just too awful to tolerate? You can avoid taking risks, up to a point. But if you do, you'll put your health and well-being at greater risk. Remember what all the studies I've mentioned add up to. If you completely avoid the risk of rejection, and don't become as connected as you need to be, you might avoid embarrassment in the short term. But the cost is steep, because in the long term you're running some far graver risks of shortening your life span.

You can't wait till you have conquered the fear of rejection to reach out. You must reach out knowing that *rejection is possible* and that *fear is part of the process*. When you do reach out despite the fear, there are many times you will get what you seek, and each of those "wins" helps to reinforce your confidence in the next encounter. That puts you ahead of the game. *People who have the courage to ask for something frequently get it.*

So, today, I ask you to *practice self-talk so you can learn to live with any reluctance you may feel*. During the previous three days, you've learned about your need to connect; you've readied some paths for making connections; and you've proven to yourself that you have the capability to get connected.

But what if you're still left with doubts that undercut your actions? Typically, those doubts come in the form of: "I don't feel I *can* do this," or "I don't think I *want* to do this."

If those tapes are playing in your head, it's time for a

conversation with yourself in which you present the positives that outweigh the negatives. That conversation may sound like this:

You: *Why don't you feel you can do this?*

Yourself: *I'm embarrassed.*

You: *Okay. Be embarrassed. But do it anyway.*

Or:

You: *Why don't you think you want to do this?*

Yourself: *I'm afraid.*

You: *Of what?*

Yourself: *I don't know.*

You: *It's okay to be afraid.*

Actually, reaching out to others can be scary. You might get rejected, after all. But you can live with the fear; it's natural and understandable and part of life. Recognize your fear—and reach out anyway.

Reach out when you think you can't, and you'll empower yourself. Maybe someone will say no when you try to connect—well, if someone does, you'll see that you can live with that rejection. Or maybe the answer will be yes, and you'll gain the rich benefits of connectedness. But you must reach.

Great things are accomplished in small steps, one step at a time. Bravery is in actually taking the step.

Results of Day 4: *You've learned how to accept the possibility of rejection.*

DAYS 5–11: THE ACTION DAYS

Over the next seven days, I am going to ask you to initiate a number of different connections. These assignments show you how many ways *you can reach beyond yourself*; in a sense, you'll be shopping for the connection that works best for you.

By the end of the week, you will have engaged with people you did not know before, will have involved yourself in your community and in a cause, will have established links to family, friends, and the life of the spirit. The more you strengthen these links in the days and months to come, the richer your life will be—and the longer your life span.

Day 5: Serve your community.

Today you must do something that will benefit your neighborhood, town, city, state, nation, or even the world.

You might start *by looking in on your neighbors.* If you have an elderly neighbor, stop by and ask whether you can bring him or her something from the supermarket. For a busy parent with preschool children, you could offer to do an errand to help out.

Call your local town hall and see if there's a volunteer hotline. Police and fire departments, for instance, often use civilian volunteers as assistants, freeing up cops and firefighters for the work they're trained to do.

During some seasons, *you can help out a local park committee.* In the spring, for instance, the group might need your help in planting bulbs or preparing garden beds. In summer, fall, or winter, there's always garden maintenance to be done.

Drop in at the library. Maybe you can help shelve books, read a story to the youngest visitors, or catalog periodicals. Is there a nearby hospital? A school? Both places put volunteers to work every day.

You might sweep the street in front of your house. Or stroll around the whole area you live in and pick up litter. Or volunteer to help out in an animal shelter.

Who can use a cup of coffee in the morning? Perhaps the school crossing guard. Or, if you live in a large apartment building, you can get a cup for the doorman.

What counts is that you step outside yourself, taking action to stay connected to your neighborhood and the world. *Devise ways that will get you out of your house and interacting with others to benefit the community.* In stepping over the threshold to do something that will make a difference to the people and place where you live, you also make a difference for yourself.

Results of Day 5: *You have initiated actions that will end your isolation and keep you connected to your community.*

Day 6: Campaign for a cause.

Quick: What's the most important issue in the world to you? The environment . . . peace . . . hunger . . . poverty . . . energy use . . . free trade . . . preservation of ancient sites . . . women's rights . . . animal welfare?

Whatever the cause or issue, today you must do something about it. Here are some possibilities:

- Write to your congressional representative about an issue that's being discussed or voted on.
- Find out about a group that's doing work you'd like to support, then donate money.
- Join a political party and ask how you can help.
- Join a committee that's taking direct action in the community.
- Campaign for animal rights.
- Get involved with a group working in the schools, neighborhood, or local government.
- If you have Internet access, search by keyword to find other resources and ideas for steps to take.

Ask yourself today what in the world you most care about. Then go on record as caring about it. Take action that expresses your concern. **Results of Day 6:** *You connect to the wider world.*

Day 7: Make a spiritual connection.

Throughout history, human beings have sensed that there is a reality beyond what can be seen and sensed in the physical realm. To many, the source of this reality is God; to others, the reality is within themselves. Wherever you find your spiritual connection, I would like you to take some time today to get in touch with it.

Connect or reconnect with the religious affiliation you grew up with. Or find another religious affiliation that may interest you. Search for your personal connection to a higher power. Think about your own sense of personal responsibility and how it guides you through your life.

Here are some of the actions you can take today to begin or restore a spiritual connection:

- Start your day with ten minutes of meditation.
- Break up your day with at least three or four moments of personal, silent prayer.
- Stop into a church, synagogue, or mosque. Spend at least a minute of silence in this place. (In any quiet sanctuary dedicated to the spirit, you are sheltered from the external world and its sights and sounds.)

Somewhere, in some form, there is something larger than yourself. And there is more to you than flesh and blood and intellect. Today, you can begin to search your religion or yourself to find it. **Results of Day 7:** *You have connected to a spirit or power that transcends yourself and your world.*

Getting the Most
from Each New Day

Not long ago, I came across some words written by Ric Kausrud a few months before his death from AIDS—what he called "a new motto for the remaining days of my life." I've kept it. Of course, none of us likes to think in terms of "remaining days," but his words say something crucial about what it means to really feel connected—not only to others, but also to the events, encounters, and surprises of every day.

This is the beginning of a new day.
I have been given this day to use as I will.
I can waste it . . . or use it for good.
But what I do today is important,
because I am exchanging a day of my life for it!
When tomorrow comes, this day will be gone forever,
leaving in its place something that I have traded for it.
I want it to be gain and not loss;
good, and not evil; success, and not failure
in order that I shall not regret the price that I have paid for it.

Day 8: Connect with the natural world.

If you live in a suburb or city, it is all too easy to forget that you are part of nature. The natural world should be a part of our lives. So today, it is time to connect again with earth and sky and the creatures that inhabit both.

What you do today may seem very simple, but most of us are so rushed that we believe we "don't have time for it." Don't be fooled by the simplicity of what you're going to do today. This is a necessary part of connecting.

Here's all you have to do.

Take a walk in the park or a nearby woods on your own. Move slowly. *Observe* carefully. *Listen* to the birds. *Reach out* and rub your hand along the bark of a tree. *Watch* the squirrels and chipmunks as they forage for food. *Smell* the roses.

If it's the dead of winter and snow covers the ground, look at the way the light plays over the top of the snow. Take a handful and look at it closely, distinguishing the separate crystals. *Feel* the cold. *Appreciate* the raw elements in which our ancestors once moved freely and easily. *Learn* to appreciate the life around you. Why wait?

If you have a whole day or part of the day off, this is a good time to call your local Audubon Society, Sierra Club, nature group, or animal shelter. Get the schedule of guided walks, and, if possible, go on one today.

Results of Day 8: *You have connected with the natural environment.*

Day 9: *Be with friends; reach out to family.*

Sometime today, I would like you to get in touch with someone who helps make you happy, encourages you, or comforts you. Friends are people who have the power to do this. There is nothing more satisfying in life than spending time with such people.

Call up a friend for a chat, meet friends for lunch, gather friends together for dinner at your home or at a restaurant.

Then *make a second call*, this time to a family member you haven't spoken to in a while. It's a link that keeps you strong.

Before the end of the day, *make an appointment* to meet with one friend or family member in the future. *Put it on your calendar* and circle the date.

Results of Day 9: *You have connected with people whose support you can rely on.*

Day 10: Join something.

In *Bowling Alone: The Collapse and Revival of American Community*, author Robert D. Putnam describes the way our connections to one another have begun to unravel over the last quarter century. The title is a reference to a phenomenon that has been observed in small towns and big cities all around the country. Bowling is a popular and usually communal recreation that millions of Americans enjoy. In recent years, the number of people who bowl has risen. But meanwhile, the number of bowling leagues and teams has declined. The point is clear—more people are bowling alone. Clearly, our community lives are less rich as a result. We are losing out on some easy opportunities to stay connected.

If you don't enjoy bowling, of course there's no reason to join a bowling league. But what other pastime do you enjoy? Where are the leagues, teams, or groups of people who enjoy the same activity?

Today, find a group to enjoy your pastime with. Have you always loved theater? If you like to participate, call the local acting group or repertory theater and find out what you can do. If acting is your thing, ask about auditions for the next show. If you prefer behind-the-scenes work, get in touch with the stage manager and find out when you can show up to paint scenery, sew costumes, or handle props.

Here are some other possibilities, depending on the focus of your interests.

- Like to sing? Inquire about a local choral group. If you belong to a church, you can join the choir. There may be a local or regional folk-music club you can join, if that's where your interest lies.

- Think it would be fun to go hiking on weekends? Join a local hiking club.
- Book clubs abound; there is one near you—and the only skill you need is the ability to read.
- Many colleges and universities have classes that are either exclusively for adults or open to auditing. Other classes are held at community colleges, arts and craft centers, and (at night) high schools. You can learn about cross-country skiing, ancient Greek, the basics of cooking, computer skills, beginning French, or how to write fiction. Today, find out about a class, short course, or lecture series that appeals to you—then sign up and join in. You'll have fun, and you'll meet people with whom you know you share at least one significant value—like you, they want to learn.

Results of Day 10: *You have connected with other people who share your interest in a subject and, like you, want to find out more.*

Day 11: Do for others.

If yesterday seemed like it was just for fun, today's assignment may turn out to be even more enjoyable. Too often we think of doing something for others as a form of serious work. True, there are few things more personally gratifying than acting in a socially responsible way. But you may be surprised at how easy, enjoyable, and immediately rewarding today's assignment turns out to be.

The assignment itself is simple: *Today, do one thing for somebody else.*

One simple way to do this is by finding a service organization in your community. Call or show up, and offer to volunteer. Most organizations welcome volunteers whatever amount of time they can give. And some will use your particular skills.

If you don't know of a local organization, call your town, county, or state government offices and ask for information about volunteer services. If you are affiliated with a religious organization that does work in homes and hospitals, call and let the organizers know that you're ready to help.

Or, if you have access to the Internet, you can log on to a wonderful site called **www.volunteermatch.org**. Just enter your zip code, and the site comes up with a list of nearby organizations that are looking for volunteers. You'll find complete information letting you know how to get in touch with the one that intrigues you. There are other Internet resources as well, so by all means do a search to find the area or organization that interests you most or where you feel you can do the greatest good.

Doing for others benefits everyone, but it pays back the doer most of all. Giving time and energy of your own free will makes you feel better, happier, and more peaceful inside—and that will make you look better on the outside. Giving a hand is one of the most strengthening actions you can take; it strengthens your connectedness to others and to the world beyond yourself, and it strengthens your chances for a longer, more fulfilling life.

Results of Day 11: *You are connected.*

Chapter 6

Day 12 and Beyond:
Replenish and Rejuvenate—
Feel Good, Look Good, Be Good to Yourself

If you've followed the four-part program of this book for the full eleven days, you've surely added at least ten years to your life. You no doubt feel better than you have in years—maybe better than you've ever felt.

You've lost weight. With exercise, you've toned up. Your clothes probably fit better, and I'll bet you feel more comfortable with your body, too. Certainly, you have eaten healthfully for eleven days. In ways that are not yet visible, your skin, eyes, hair, and teeth are already getting the benefits of your improved health.

But here's the other benefit of this program—the difference that it makes in your appearance.

Personally, I can see the difference immediately in patients when they get a handle on stress. And it's even more apparent when people make connections with others and with the world around them. Now that you're in charge of your life and attuned to your community, I'll bet you don't have that worried look anymore. When someone appears stooped over, or looks away from other people, it's as if they're trying to hide from the world. You don't have to do that—do you? Instead, you're now stepping up to life, shoulders back, visage open to the world, ready to engage, much more confident. It's a better way to look.

The Wow Factor

Before long, your friends and colleagues will notice. I call it the Wow Factor: "Wow. You look great. What have you done?" It's exciting to hear, and it's an exciting way to feel.

Of course, as the four-part program of this book becomes a way of life, dramatic changes will diminish. You'll still feel good, and you'll still look good, but now the issue will become how to keep the Wow Factor alive—how to maintain that wonderful new look forever and how to keep on feeling as terrific as you do today.

The answer is pretty simple: Be good to yourself. Treat yourself as lovingly and as generously as you would treat anyone you love. Pamper yourself. You deserve some luxuries. Remember that too much of a good thing is an awfully good thing.

You've taken care of the beauty within by learning to manage your stress, by undertaking regular physical activity, by changing your relationship with food, and by reaching out to the wider world. *You've given yourself the great gift of a longer and better life. Now it's time to ensure that you always look the part.*

The Spa Treatment— Not to Be Missed!

If you're wondering how to treat yourself very well, let me make a strong recommendation. A spa is a great place to start.

There are now thousands of spas in the United States and Mexico. You can easily find one that fits your taste, and at some, the costs are quite reasonable. At a destination spa, you can stay for as long as you like—from a day to two weeks, or longer. But there are also day spas. In just a few hours at a day spa, you get a quick "hit" of pampering. You can focus on the services you need or enjoy the most, then return home refreshed—feeling as if you've been away much longer!

In general, there are three types of spas: those focusing on health and fitness, those focusing on spiritual harmony and relaxation, and those that combine both approaches.

Health and fitness spas feature health-enhancing programs, lectures and education, cardio training, diet and weight-loss programs, as well as exercise.

Spas that focus on the spiritual generally offer programs in yoga, tai chi, chi kung, and meditation. The pampering treatments are holistic, and the spas will feature wellness consultations and bodywork. You can get muscle-soothing massage, sign up for antiaging programs, and explore rejuvenation treatments for body and face.

At a *"combo spa"* you can address health and fitness problems like weight loss and stress management while also following the holistic approach of a spiritual/relaxation spa. The *Canyon Ranch* spa, a trendsetter, is one of the leading examples of this kind of spa.

All spas offer healthful cuisine, and all feature a range of treatments for skin wellness, hand and foot care, facials, body treatments, and massage.

What's a Spa Treatment Like?

If you've already visited a destination spa, you know what it's like (and I'm sure you're looking forward to your next visit!). If you haven't, here is a sampling of what you can expect at a couple of destination spas at the southern tip of Mexico's Baja Peninsula—the famed Las Ventanas resort in Los Cabos and Sueños del Mar Spa at the Casa del Mar resort in Cabo San Lucas.

Las Ventanas is well known as a celebrity hangout. Rated one of the top three spas in the world, it's renowned for its Desert Signature Treatments. Everything about the place is geared to appeal to the senses. The grounds are perfectly landscaped. Gardens are exquisite, and from them come the even more exquisite floral arrangements that grace the interior. The very architecture of the buildings invites you into an experience of unparalleled luxury.

You can enjoy a voluptuous lifestyle at Las Ventanas. At poolside, attendants will clean your sunglasses, spray your tanning body with cool mineral water, and keep you constantly supplied with ice water with lemon. The elegant and superb light spa cuisine—served in one of the five restaurants, on the beach, or in your own suite—focuses on regional flavors. For exercise or relaxation, try yachting, windsurfing, marine wildlife expeditions, golf, tennis, sailing, or an excursion across the Baja desert.

Afterward, treat yourself to one of Las Ventanas' famed spa treatments, many of them performed outside in the sweet Baja air. Maybe you've just enjoyed a round of golf or a tough bout of windsurfing. It's a good time to try the *analgesic muscle relaxer*. First, your skin is thoroughly cleansed with a loofah scrub of antioxidant and analgesic herbs; then comes a delightful shower; finally, you get a sports massage in which those same analgesic herbs are used to soothe pain and wake up tired muscles.

Or how about the *sea enzyme body wrap with green tea and*

ginger? It takes eighty minutes. At the beginning of the treatment, you'll be given a detoxifying body scrub with a mixture of grape seeds, papaya, and pineapple. Afterward, you'll get a body mask of green tea, gingerroot, and seaweed, followed by a wrap and facial massage—all aimed at releasing tension, balancing energy, and replenishing vitamins and minerals.

Another delicious eighty-minute treatment is the *gentlemen's facial*—deep cleansing, purifying, and relaxing. This is followed by a scalp massage and, finally, a foot reflexology treatment.

Then there's the *therapeutic antioxidant treatment*, the *European aromatherapy facial*, or maybe the *thermal anti-cellulite treatment*. Feeling a little muscle pain? A good remedy is Austrian moor mud—rich, creamy mud from Vorarlberg, Austria, containing a thousand herbs, organic substances, and trace elements that purify the lymph system, tone skin, stimulate circulation, and help relieve muscle pain. Even arthritis pain can be eased with this treatment. Or perhaps you'd prefer *raindrop therapy, a full-body massage that boosts the immune system, releases muscle spasms, and lowers inflammation.* It's given outdoors on the beach, just steps from the Pacific.

Not far away on the peninsula is the cozy *Casa del Mar resort* in Cabo San Lucas, where you'll find the Sueños del Mar Spa with a similar bounty of offerings. There, you might want to start your stay by exfoliating away all the tired "stuff" you've been accumulating onto your skin. Spend seventy-five minutes getting the *tropical exfoliation*, in which a combination of ground coffee beans and dried coconut is applied all over, preparing your skin for tanning. The session ends with a massage.

Or you might prefer the *chocolate and mint escape, an hour and a half of chocolate exfoliation, a chocolate and mint massage, and a cup of hot cocoa to warm you inside.* When you're not being pampered by the very attentive staff at Casa del Mar, try horseback riding, kayaking, scuba diving, or snorkeling in the crystal clear Sea of Cortez.

Got the picture? In a two-day visit or a two-week splurge, you can feel your body and soul rejuvenated and very nearly reborn at a spa.

Your Own Home Spa

You don't have to go to a spa to approximate the kind of voluptuous treatments it offers or the environment it represents. In a suburban house or city apartment, you don't have expert masseurs and fitness professionals dedicated to giving you first-rate treatment in a luxury setting. But many of the components of an equally satisfying spa treatment are easily within reach.

When you consider the simple elements of spa care, what do you have? In nearly all spas, you'll get body treatments, hand and foot care, skin care, hair and scalp treatments, and facials. In luxurious spas, all this takes place in a relaxing environment where you can get into a deliciously self-indulgent mood. And yet even without the luxury environment—even if you never leave home— you can create the right environment for luxurious self-care.

Start by creating a spa-like atmosphere using household items and the principles of aromatherapy. Set scented candles around your bathroom—even on the tub. Dim the lights. In a nearby room, put on some soothing music—just loud enough to set the mood, not loud enough to sing along to. Run a warm bath and put in ten drops of essential oils or bath salts.

If what you want is a relaxing, calming bath, use lavender, bergamot, or cedarwood. If you want an energizing bath, try lemon, rosemary, or frankincense.

Get into the tub. Soothe yourself down into it. Let the water cover your body.

While you're soaking, put a deep-conditioning mask on your clean hair, then wrap your head in a plastic wrap or a shower cap. You can make your own conditioning mask by mixing essential oils like chamomile (if your hair is light) or rosemary (for dark hair) with an egg, lanolin, and glycerin. (Lanolin and glycerin are available at most drugstores.)

After a long soak, polish your skin with an exfoliating scrub. I recommend a scrub containing walnut shells, apricot kernels, or fine granular pumice, which work best to remove dead skin cells. The scrubs are available at many fine department stores as well as pharmacies and skin-care stores. Apply the scrub gently with a loofah, brush, or sponge. Rinse yourself well—washing away all that dead skin—then get out of the tub. Exchange the shower cap for a towel turban on your hair to keep in the warmth and to enhance the conditioning effects.

As you pat your body dry, be sure to leave some moisture on your skin. Finish up with your favorite body lotion, rubbing in that excess moisture so it stays "trapped" on your skin.

More Spa-style Care at Home

While you're in your home-spa environment, try a foot scrub or use a pumice stone to clean any calluses. Then moisturize your feet with an invigorating foot cream. Peppermint is a great choice.

Use a skin pad to buff the insides of both palms. Moisturize your hands with your favorite lotion and slip them into an old pair of cotton gloves. Take a heating pad and place it over the palms of the hands for five to ten minutes. Then turn your hands over and return the heating pad to the tops of your hands for five to ten minutes. This enhances moisturization.

Do all this, and you'll go back to your day job just about as refreshed and just about as pampered as if you had come from the most luxurious spa on earth.

Your Skin-deep Beauty

There's one more thing you can do to keep yourself feeling and looking as good as possible for your entire life—and that's taking care of your skin.

Signs of aging show up first in the skin. Tissue simply breaks down as we get older. Collagen becomes depleted. If you've spent a lot of time in the sun, the frequent exposure begins to take its toll.

Have you ever smoked? That habit pulls moisture from your skin.

Are you a regular drinker of morning coffee? That can also deplete moisture, as can the evening cocktail.

From without and within, free radical scavengers that damage cellular structure do their work, and skin that was once smooth and supple begins to sag and wrinkle.

By following the eleven-day Picture Perfect Prescription, you've already done a lot to counteract the natural aging process of the skin. *By learning to manage your stress*, for example, you've put a stop to one of the major causes of premature skin aging, for stress increases the free radicals in the body that damage skin, even as it exacerbates such skin conditions as hives, rosacea, acne, and cold sores. *By starting to exercise regularly*, you're improving skin tone and fighting the natural breakdown of skin's building blocks.

By eating well—and especially by avoiding high-calorie foods and greasy, fatty foods and adding more fresh fruits and vegetables—you're helping keep skin tissue healthy and rich in nutrients.

Best Foods for Skin Care

Some foods can directly affect your skin. Check out the Picture Perfect Prescription Food Pyramid on page 149. Everything in its Fats and Oils rung can help counteract skin drying or flakiness. The selenium in seafood and whole grains, the beta-carotene and vitamins in root vegetables and citrus fruits, and the vitamins found in seeds and nuts deactivate damaging free radicals and keep skin looking and feeling fresh. So by continuing to eat the pyramid way, you'll also be doing your skin a big favor.

Even *reaching out to others* can help keep your skin young, for it contributes to that overall sense of well-being that is reflected in healthy skin.

Complementing and supplementing all this good news is the

special care you can give your skin now. Your skin gets that special care whenever you take a home-spa bath, or use topical treatments that help your skin fight damaging free radicals and give a boost to your body's own natural antioxidants. But best of all is the at-home facial.

Looking Younger All the Time

Experts recommend two types of regular skin care for your face. *Give yourself a daily facial,* they advise, and *at least once a month, supplement that facial with a steaming and a mask application.*

The basic facial includes three steps: *cleanse, exfoliate,* and *moisturize.*

Before you begin, wash your hands. (You don't want to transfer bacteria and dirt from hands to face.) Then take the following steps:

1. *Cleanse.* Use a gentle cleanser to wash your face and neck. To make your own cleanser, use milk with a little olive oil. Massage it well into the skin. Use a circular motion and massage upward from the neck.

2. *Exfoliate.* When the face is well cleansed, begin the exfoliation. This will strip off the top layer of dead skin cells and will leave fresh skin. Use over-the-counter exfoliating scrubs containing a variety of ingredients that will gently remove dirt and dead cells, unclog pores, and correct the damage done by free-radical scavengers. (You can also make your own exfoliant: combine oatmeal, crushed almonds or almond oil, and mint for an added

energizing effect; add a little water to make a paste.) After gently rubbing the exfoliant into the skin, rinse it off and pat your face dry. This polishing effect leaves skin clean, smooth, and silky.

Whichever exfoliant you use, be gentle: use careful, gentle motions, avoid the eye area, and do not use on irritated or broken-out skin. You will find that even if your face has begun to wrinkle, the cleansing and exfoliation will decrease the appearance of aging.

3. *Moisturize.* Moisturizing creams can seal moisture onto the skin. For this hydrating process to occur, be sure you don't entirely dry the skin after rinsing; let the moisture sink in, then apply the moisturizing cream as a coating.

You can choose from among a range of facial moisturizers. Look for topicals that bring back the natural properties of your skin that aging and the environment have depleted. You want natural ingredients, both common and exotic, that can replenish your skin.

One or two times a month—but not more often—*add a steaming process and a mask treatment after exfoliation and before moisturizing.* For a facial steaming, pour boiling water into a large bowl, adding herbs, green tea, or lemon juice. (If you have particularly sensitive skin, apply a thin layer of moisturizer before you steam. This will keep your skin from becoming irritated.) Hold your cleansed face a comfortable distance above the bowl. Using a towel to make a tent over your head, just let the steam rise into your face.

Let your skin "drink in" the steam for about five minutes. This softens the top layer of skin, and you can then *finish off your facial with a moisturizer—or proceed to the mask treatment.*

For the mask treatment, you want a mask designed especially for your skin type. If your skin is sensitive, choose something soothing that has a chamomile base. If your skin is oily, rosemary or sage is recommended. For normal skin, try lavender or rose.

Want to make your own mask? Try either of these mixtures:

• an egg yolk with honey and safflower oil

• yellow cornmeal or oatmeal with honey

Both combinations work well to tighten the pores. Add plain yogurt to brighten your skin. (You might also add aloe if available, although it is not necessary.)

Make a paste, keep it on your face and neck for fifteen minutes, rinse it off, and pat dry. Be sure to leave the skin a bit moist. Then moisturize.

On the horizon are unique formulations using state-of-the-art technology that will be a Picture Perfect Prescription creating a picture-perfect face.

In all cases, when you care for your face—or your hands, feet, hair, body, or soul—do it gently and with love. *Defy age. Be good to yourself. You deserve it.*

Resources

Move

Fred DeVito, core fusion
http://exhalespa.com: click on Mind Body Classes, then click on
Core Fusion

Ron Fletcher, Pilates
www.ronfletcherwork.com

DVD's
Fletcher Spine Corrector™
Pilates Matwork
Fletcher Towelwork™

Michael Lechonczak, yoga
www.intelligentyoga.com

Book
Consultant on *Real Men Do Yoga: 21 Star Athletes Reveal Their*

Secrets for Strength, Flexibility and Peak Performance by John Capouya, HCI, 2003

Heather Raymond, personal trainer
superwomanhr@aol.com

Lawrence Tan, martial arts
www.tandao.com

Book
Universal Form: Three-Minute Routine for Transforming Stress to Power and Peace, by Lawrence Tan, Shambhala Press, 1998

Videos
The Universal Form, Three Minutes to Power and Peace, Wellspring Media

Yamuna Zake, bodyrolling
http://www.yamunabodyrolling.com/

Books
The Ultimate Body Rolling Workout: The Revolutionary Way to Tone, Lengthen, and Realign Your Body by Yamuna Zake and Stephanie Golden, Broadway Books, 2003

Body Rolling: An Experiential Approach to Complete Muscle Release by Yamuna Zake and Stephanie Golden, Healing Art Press, 1997

Videos
Total Body Workout, Sideline, Foot Saver, Abdominal Routine, YBR Anywhere, Leg Routine

Eat

www.drhowardshapiro.com
www.pictureperfectweightloss.com

Books
Dr. Shapiro's Picture Perfect Weight Loss
Picture Perfect Weight Loss Shopper's Guide
Picture Perfect Weight Loss Thirty Day Plan
Picture Perfect Weight Loss Cookbook

Connect

http://www.assistanceleague.org/home2.cfm
www.volunteermatch.org

Replenish and Rejuvenate

http://www.lasventanas.com/
http://www.mexonline.com/casamar.htm
http://www.canyonranch.com/
www.posnercosmetics.com

References

p.3. L. Hayflick, "The Future of Aging," *Nature*, 408 (2000): 267–9.

p.29. Glaser, Ronald, Ph.D. Department of Medical Microbiology and Immunology, Behavioral Medicine Research Institute, Ohio State University Health Sciences Center
Summary of presentation December 17, 1996, Science Writers Briefing sponsored by the OBSSR and the American Psychological Association.

p. 41. BlueCross BlueShield Health Care Center of Greater New York, stress pamphlet.

p.56. Edited from *The American Heritage Dictionary of the English Language*, third edition, copyright © 1992 by Houghton Mifflin Company. Electronic version licensed from INSO Corporation. All rights reserved.

pp.137–38. Statistics from U.S. Surgeon General and from study of 3,457 middle-aged population in Framingham, Massachusetts (Framingham Heart Study). Reported in www.weight-loss-i.com/weight-lifespan-longevity.htm.

pp.137–38. Compiled by Nutritional Management, Inc., 990 Washington Street, Suite 211S, Dedham, MA 02026.

p.208. Erich, Fromm, *Escape from Freedom*, 1941.

p. 210. http://vanderbiltowc.wellsource.com/dh/content_print.asp?ID=563

p.225. New York, Simon & Schuster, 2000.

Credits

COMPANION DVD

Part 1:

Picture This: Weight Loss with Dr. Howard Shapiro

This segment is from *Picture This: Weight Loss with Dr. Howard Shapiro*

Produced by Connecticut Public Television (CPTV)

Distributed nationally by American Public Television (APT)

Producer: Harriet Unger

Connecticut Public Television

240 New Britain Avenue

Hartford, CT 06106

1-860-278-5310

Website: www.cptv.org/TVNationalShapiro.asp

Copyright 2001 CPTV

Part 2:

All segments are produced and copyrighted by Chamberlain Bros. 2005, except for Pilates with Ron Fletcher.

COMPANION CD

Part 1:

Recipes TXT file, all recipes copyright 2005 Dr. Howard Shapiro.

Part 2:

Calorie Calculator - Calories Burned, BMI, BMR & RMR Calculator*

Courtesy www.caloriesperhour.com

Copyright 2000-2004

For more information on BMI, BMR, RMR, Kilojoules, Calories, or any other information regarding the site and their calculations, go to www.caloriesperhour.com.

Sources for calculator include, but are not limited to:

Except as noted below, the METs used to calculate the number of calories burned are adapted from Ainsworth BE, Haskell WL, Whitt MC, Irwin ML, Swartz AM, Strath SJ, O'Brien WL, Bassett DR Jr, Schmitz KH, Emplaincourt PO, Jacobs DR Jr, Leon AS. Compendium of Physical Activities: An update of activity codes and MET intensities. Med Sci Sports Exerc 2000;32 (Suppl):S498-S516.

The following list indicates sources other than the Compendium of Physical Activities:

In-Line Skating: Calculations for calories burned for in-line skating are not based on METs as are calculations for other activities. The calculator uses an equation developed by Bob Kalish. The equation is based on the data presented in the chart at rollerblade.com.

Pilates: METs were estimated by Kevin Bowen, President and Co-founder of Pilates Method Alliance, by comparing Pilates to activities listed in the Compendium.

Snowboarding: METs were estimated based on the results of the calculator at self.com.

Tae Bo: METs were estimated based on Billy Blanks estimation that Tae Bo burns between 800 and 1200 calories per hour depending on workout intensity and other variables.

TreadClimber: METs were taken from a study conducted by Adelphi University.

Treadmill: MET readings were taken from the console of a popular treadmill.

Part 3:
Life Expectancy Calculator

The information and materials appearing on the attached website pages are presented for your personal, non-commercial use only. They may not be reproduced, duplicated or distributed without written permission from either www.caloriesperhour.com or www.livingto100.com. Copying these materials for anything other than your personal use is a violation of United States copyright laws. Penguin Group (USA) Inc. makes no warranties, express or implied, about the information and materials appearing on these websites, which is provided "as is." Penguin Group (USA) Inc. will not be responsible for third party materials on either website. If you access this material outside the US you are responsible for compliance with local laws. Neither www.caloriesperhour.com nor www.livingto100.com make no warranties, express or implied, about the information and materials appearing in PICTURE PERFECT PRESCRIPTION BY Dr. Howard Shapiro, which is provided "as is."